All of us who have in whatever way come into contact with the Hemi-Sync process are indebted to its discoverer and developer, Robert Monroe. Without his courage, persistence, and unique overview, our world would be a poorer place. With the love and admiration of its editor and contributors, this book is dedicated to him.

— USING THE —
WHOLE
BRAIN

Integrating the Right and Left Brain With Hemi-Sync Sound Patterns

Edited by
Ronald Russell

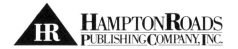
HAMPTONROADS
PUBLISHING COMPANY, INC.

For information write:

Hampton Roads Publishing Company, Inc.
891 Norfolk Square
Norfolk, VA 23502

Or call: (804)459-2453
FAX: (804)455-8907

If you are unable to order this book from your local
bookseller, you may order directly from the publisher.
Quantity discounts for organizations are available.
Call 1-800-766-8009, toll-free.

ISBN 1-878901-86-9

Printed on acid-free paper in the United States of America

Contents

Applications: Mind

Applications: Spirit

Applications: Scientific and Technical

Outreach

Addenda

Preface
The Way of Hemi-Sync

The inescapable Law of Cause and Effect can't be ignored, whatever the situation or the reaction. We may or may not like or anticipate the result. Yet there will be one even many years later. That is the case in Hemi-Sync, our acronym for hemispheric synchronization. Back in 1956, our New York-based company had been a leader in the production of radio network programs, using voices, music, and specialized sound. With the rising power of television, a decision had to be made whether to convert to this new medium or to try something else.

A possibility came to our attention: learning during sleep, that third of our lives over which we had little or no control and where much of our time and energy may well be wasted.

We set up a Research & Development program to explore the prospect and immediately ran into the basic problem. We couldn't get our subjects to go to sleep when we needed them to do so for test periods. The use of sleep-inducing drugs seemed contradictory to our basic purpose.

Using our area of expertise, we began testing subjects with various sound patterns to find those that would evoke various stages of sleep. It was slow work, but we did have just enough early success to lure us to continue.

When EEG testing of subjects showed waveforms similar if not identical to the sound patterns we were using, we began to call the result Frequency Following Response (FFR). Later, as we began using binaural beat sound, we found similar waveforms in both sides of the brain at the same moment. This brain hemispheric synchronization came to be known as Hemi-Sync.

I had been one of the leading subjects in our tests. In 1958, I began to experience states of consciousness totally unknown to me. They seemed both dangerous and exciting. Other subjects did not experience the phenomenon. As a result, we diverted our research into this new area.

Through the years, our work progressed steadily in this seemingly new direction, attracting the attention, interest, and participation of several hundred researchers, scientists, engineers, educators, physicians, psychologists, and many others. They are the ones, not I, who have brought the Hemi-Sync processes to the level they are today. I am still not sure I was the sole cause.

The effects? Over 200,000 people now have a good night's sleep without drugs, as a baseline. Many thousands more have learned better understanding and control of their mental, emotional, and physical selves. We believe it is an emerging learning system that might be called **Lifespan,** applicable from cradle to grave.

Thus the purpose of this volume is to acquaint you with the various practical applications of the Hemi-Sync process, so that you also will begin to consider how you can make use of it, not only in your personal life but in many other areas as well.

> Robert A. Monroe
> The Monroe Institute

Acknowledgements

My thanks are due to all those who so generously provided contributions for this book and also to those for whose contributions there was insufficient space. I am grateful also to Leslie France, Shirley Bliley, Darlene Miller, Ron Harris, and those others of the staff of The Monroe Institute who gave assistance where and when it was needed. F. Holmes (Skip) Atwater, the Institute's Executive Director, and Mark Certo, sound engineer, provided valuable advice on the more technical aspects of the Hemi-Sync process. The editorial task was lightened by the aid, comfort, and sustenance so kindly provided by Eleanor Friede. To Jill, who encouraged and assisted this undertaking and whose advice I should always accept— and usually do—I am eternally grateful.

Introduction

Consciousness is something that we all share. Yet its nature and its potential remain, by and large, a mystery. We still know very little about how sensory perception leads to awareness and how ideas come into being. We have very little understanding about our feelings or the ways in which our attitudes affect our perception and behavior. And the self, that most intimate aspect of the conscious mind, remains as mysterious as ever. This may be the next great frontier. Its exploration could lead to a wealth of "inner technologies" concerned not with managing matter or information, but with the management of our own minds.
Peter Russell,
The White Hole in Time (Harper, 1992)

It was in the early 1970s, after more than a decade of research, that one of these "inner technologies" made its first appearance in a laboratory in the depths of rural Virginia. Here a small group headed by a former radio executive and sound engineer, Robert Monroe, worked to implement a vision—in the words of Nancy McMoneagle, the coordinator of the group, "to explore, develop, and give practical application to expanded states of consciousness in order to bring something of value to contemporary culture." In 1979 the group, now known as The Monroe Institute, moved to Nelson County, Virginia, where a residential center for programs, a laboratory, a conference center, and administrative offices were built on wooded hills a few miles east of the Blue Ridge Mountains.

In the following years, training courses in the development of consciousness were established and refined. Word-of-mouth reports and Monroe's widely read book, *Journeys Out of the Body*, brought inquiries and course participants from all over the world. Research continued energetically, and the Institute found its place on the leading edge of investigation into human consciousness. A Professional Division, consisting of members who used the Institute's technology in their professional work, was established, and in 1985

13

The Monroe Institute became a non-profit organization. In 1987 a brainmapping research project was launched, and new programs inviting participants to probe more deeply into consciousness were introduced. Experts in many areas and from many countries came to find out what was going on, to contribute their own experience, and to provide their own input.

Monroe's initial discovery, on which the research, programs, and products of the Institute are based, was that "certain patterns of sound will induce distinct states of consciousness not ordinarily available to the human mind." Investigation into specific sound combinations and frequencies is continuous, and methods and techniques have been developed so that the mind patterns created by the sounds may be maintained and controlled by the individual. Users of the technology, therefore, learn conscious control of many different and productive states of consciousness. The Educational Division of the Institute conducts classes and seminars and disseminates audio tapes and other materials in direct application of the methods it has researched. The process that the Institute has developed is known and registered as Hemi-Sync, an abbreviation of Hemispheric Synchronization. The hemispheres are those of the human cerebral cortex. While as far as is known neither hemisphere has a monopoly of any given function, research has shown that each appears to be dominant in particular areas. Here are some examples:

Left	Right
Speech	Voice intonation
Logic	Emotion
Reason	Intuition
Temporal	Spatial
Objective	Subjective
Rhythm	Melody, pitch
Time sense (past, present, future)	Present-oriented
Directed	Spontaneous

In addition, Ornstein and Sobel (*The Healing Brain*, 1988) declare that ". . .on EEG and recognition measures, emotions like anger and sadness involve the right hemisphere more than the left, while emotions like happiness involve the left hemisphere."

Our educational systems in the West nurture left-hemisphere dominance; indeed, we might suggest that Western civilization is essentially left-brain dominant, while older, tribal civilizations are (or were) right-brain dominant. But we must always bear in mind that in making suggestions of this sort we are grossly simplifying what is very complex and still imperfectly understood.

The Hemi-Sync process seeks to produce in the listener whole-brain coherence, a state of consciousness defined when the electroencephalograph (EEG) patterns of both hemispheres are simultaneously equal in amplitude and frequency. This, it seems, rarely happens in normal everyday life, and when it does it lasts for only a very short time. It is possible for an experienced meditator to achieve and maintain this state for some minutes; Elmer and Alyce Green, pioneers of Biofeedback, discovered when researching at the Menninger Foundation that a subject with twenty years of training in Zen meditation could establish this synchronized state at will and sustain it for more than fifteen minutes. The audio techniques developed at The Monroe Institute are able to induce and sustain this state in the listener in the very first exercise undertaken.

What is the value of this state of whole-brain coherence? Patricia Carrington, of Princeton University, expresses it thus:

> Man's highest achievements obviously require the complementary workings of thought processes from both sides of the brain. Intuition and hunches must be shaped through logical, disciplined thinking to form a work of art, and the most rigorous scientific and philosophic reasoning requires the enriching leaven of hunch and inspiration. We need a harmony, a coming together of our two "selves" into one mind. (*Handbook of States of Consciousness*, ed. B.B. Wolman & M. Ullman, p.487 *et seq.*)

The process which seeks to produce this coherence is based on two naturally occurring auditory phenomena: frequency following response (FFR) and binaural ("two-ears") beat stimulation. The frequency following response is essentially a process of entrainment. When you listen closely to sounds of specific frequencies, you tend to reproduce those frequencies in your own physiology. Furthermore, you can become entrained to the state of awareness engendered by those frequencies (for example, they can alert you, relax you, or send you to sleep). In time, you can learn to reproduce this state of awareness at will, without the audio stimulation. The tapes on which the signals are recorded are just training wheels; you discard them when you can manage to make these "consciousness shifts" on your own.

Binaural beats are produced within your physiology when different audio frequencies are introduced into each ear. The brain discerns this difference and seeks to bridge the gap. In so doing, it produces a third frequency—the difference between the two. This is not an actual sound, although you may be aware of an oscillating or wavering note. For example, if a sound of 100 Hz (cycles per second) is introduced into one ear and one of 104 Hz into the other, the binaural beat frequency will be 4 Hz. The human ear cannot detect a sound of such low frequency; 40 Hz is about our limit. The binaural beat system, therefore, provides the opportunity for a listener to be influenced by frequencies below the threshold of normal human hearing. Moreover, it tends to stimulate a state of low-frequency brain-wave interhemispheric synchronization. Results of this synchrony include an amplification in the attention a listener is able to apply while in a targeted state of awareness. The binaural beat stimulation makes it possible to sustain this focus of attention over relatively long periods of time.

However, it should be noted that the strength and uniqueness of Hemi-Sync is not simply that it employs binaural beats or makes use of the frequency following response. Its advantage lies in the precisely identified wave forms, blended and sequenced over time into specific, complex frequency patterns. It is a process; a combination of multiplexed audio binaural beats and pink sound, verbal suggestion, amplified placebo effect, relaxation exercises, guided imagery, and autohypnosis, all carefully crafted to engender desired mental states of consciousness. It does not employ any subliminal suggestions.

The Monroe Institute works with beat frequencies mostly in what are known as the beta, alpha, theta, and delta ranges; that is, from 30 Hz to 0.5 Hz. Certain combinations of frequencies have been identified as conducive to stimulating particular mind-brain states (for example, concentration, deep relaxation, enhanced learning). The process quickly guides you into a targeted, sustained state of awareness within which you are able to apply a unique focus of attention toward achieving your desired outcome. The process guides you; it does not compel you. Your response is always under your own control. In brief, Hemi-Sync is a self-controlled tool that enables its users to accomplish their own goals by facilitating and sustaining a purposefully focused, highly productive, coherent mind-brain state.

How does it feel to be in a state of complete brain hemispheric synchronization? It resembles that type of meditative state when you are physically fully relaxed with the mind open and alert. This state may be seen as a starting point, or a gateway through which you may move into areas untroubled by physical sensory input, unrestricted by time and space. In these areas you may use left brain methodology—the intellectual, analytical part of the mind—to explore the right brain—the intuitive, emotional, visuo-spatial territories. As Robert Monroe says:

> All of the Institute's training systems without exception, whether 'live' or on tape, are nothing less than surrogate 'left-brain' devices that enable the user/participant to hold on to his analytical capability during unusual and exotic states of consciousness. Thus they permit growth through familiarity and understanding, and work on the greatest barrier of all—fear.

There are a few terms used in the Hemi-Sync exercises, and in some of the articles that follow, to describe certain brain states. They are listed below in the order in which the states are attained in the Institute's teaching programs.

C1 (Consciousness 1): Everyday "normal" waking consciousness.

Focus 3: A state where the brain and mind are more coherent, synchronized, and balanced than in everyday consciousness.

Focus 10: Hemispheric synchronization. Body asleep (to all intents and purposes), mind awake and alert. Deep physical relaxation combined with mental alertness.

Focus 12: A state of expanded awareness. A "high energy" state in which one becomes more conscious of inner resources and guidance.

Focus 15: Time as a construct of consciousness no longer exists.

Focus 21: A state in which one may move freely into other energy systems.

Professional and practical work is undertaken using Focus 3, 10 and 12. Work in Focus 15 and 21 is confined to courses at the Institute, and Focus 22 to 27 are explored in the Lifeline course.

In the following chapters we look at some of the practical applications of the Hemi-Sync technology. Many of the contributions originate from members of the Institute's Professional Division reporting on their work with clients, patients, and students. Others come from people who have experienced the benefits themselves—who have undergone the surgery or the dentistry or have their own stories to tell. Some contributions have previously appeared in the Institute's own publications, *Focus, Breakthrough,* and *Hemi-Sync Journal;* some are adapted from books shortly to be published or from other journals; some have been transcribed from talks or lectures; while the remainder have been specially written for this volume. In all, they provide a wide-ranging survey of the practical uses and applications of the Monroe technology.

There is no suggestion that this technology is a panacea for all ills or meets with success every time it is used. What is especially interesting, however, is that so few negative comments are reported; there are no side effects and no danger of addiction. On the few occasions when adverse comments have been made, it has almost always been found that the tapes were played too loudly, and reducing the volume has made them acceptable. Michael Hutchison, an investigative journalist who conducted a series of trials of various tools and techniques for brain growth and mind expansion for his book *Megabrain,* says, "I did not encounter anyone who had a negative response to the Hemi-Sync experience."

Since its inception, the Institute has been generous in sharing its discoveries and has withstood the competition of a number of heavily advertised look-alike systems and samples of hardware—the Institute has always refrained from mass advertising of its products. While public interest in phenomena such as channelling, out-of-body experiences, spontaneous healing, aura reading, and so on has blossomed, the Institute has maintained its scientific, investigative approach, all the while challenging limiting belief systems, whether "Old" or "New" Age in origin.

In the past, however, the scientific community, wherever and whenever it has heard of Hemi-Sync, has tended to dismiss it as a temporary fad, another "New Age" fashion with no real basis, or at best as a technique which may have a psychological but not a physiological effect. It may be that this dismissive approach has denied the benefits of the process to numbers of people in pain or suffering from stress-related conditions, anxious, tense, unrelaxed, unhappy, for whom only a course of medical drugs could be prescribed. Orthodox medicine, with its current reliance on expensive technology, understandably finds it difficult to give credence to such a cheap and simple device as an audio cassette tape as a substitute for a costly course of medication or heavy dose of anesthetic. Those practitioners who are prepared to swim against the tide, who are willing to use these taped exercises with their patients without waiting years for long and expensive series of double-blind tests meticulously reported in acceptable medical journals, are brave indeed. Yet their bravery is rewarded by the progress of their patients— see Gari Carter's story in Chapter 2 for a moving example of this.

Perhaps the tide is beginning to turn. Fashion in medicine, as in other areas, is subject to change. Doctors such as Bernie Siegel, Larry Dossey, Art Gladman (an advisor to The Monroe Institute), and Elisabeth Kubler-Ross (a Monroe course participant) show their awareness, and demonstrate in their own work, that man is not just a collection of diseases, a case of cancer or a bowel complaint, but a whole person and much more than just his physical body. The great importance of the mind in the healing process is more and more becoming acknowledged. As Ornstein and Sobel point out, it is "the belief in the remedy and in the healer (or in something else) that seems to have mobilized powerful innate self-healing mechanisms within the brain." Strong belief heals, they say; and belief in the efficacy of the Monroe process, based on the knowledge that Hemi-Sync works, may lead to its playing an ever more important part in the medicine of the future.

Is it possible to sum up the benefits of Hemi-Sync in a sentence or two? Not altogether; each person's experience is unique and each response may be subtly different. After his trials, Michael Hutchison collected comments from participants on the changes in consciousness they had experienced. These included: intense mental clarity; dramatic reductions of chronic pain (from several sufferers of arthritis, lower back pain and migraine headaches); deep meditation; sudden flashes of insight or "eureka!" moments; euphoria; profound relaxation; lucid dreaming; peak experiences; and out-of-body experiences. To these we can add: reduction of anxiety; enhanced creativity and a breaking down of "writer's block"; increased appreciation of nature; and a generally heightened awareness that seems to be permanent.

On a purely "everyday" level, Hemi-Sync may help you improve your sporting abilities, in particular tennis or golf. The technology may enable you to overcome addictive habits, such as smoking, and its use can provide an environment for creative thinking and decision-making in business life. In addition, the Human Plus series of exercises conveys a means of bringing the power of the mind to bear on a wide range of physical and emotional conditions, reminding us that if we cease to treat mind and body as separate entities our problems will more easily be solved.

And this is only part of the story. There are several thousand people who have attended courses at the Institute and many thousands more who have taken part in weekend training workshops or who have used the taped exercises in their own homes. If all that happens is that through moving into different states of awareness they get to know themselves rather better, then the experience for that alone has been worth while and its value is confirmed. But in most instances this is by no means all that happens. One workshop participant speaks for many when she says "I've been recommending Monroe tapes to various friends as I do feel they've helped me so much—not only in helping me relax but also in contacting inner wisdom to guide one through the turbulence of everyday existence."

In the following chapters are many examples of the life-changing experiences that individuals have reported. What is common here is a strengthening of the sense of self-worth, an increased confidence, the knowledge—not just the belief—that one is able to transcend one's supposed limitations. In this process there is no dogma; no guru instructs you; no beliefs are imposed. To Robert Monroe, begetter of the system, Kahlil Gibran's concept of a teacher (in *The Prophet*) fittingly applies: "If he is indeed wise, he does not bid you enter the house of his wisdom, but rather leads you to the threshold of your own mind."

Commenting on the "inner technologies" concerned with the management of our minds that he sees emerging, Peter Russell says:

> They are likely to be techniques and processes that assist our mental functioning—help us think more clearly, remember better, clarify our perception, feel more fully, free ourselves from fear, release our creativity, communicate more clearly and relate more honestly. They will be technologies that bring greater mastery of our minds, a greater awareness of our selves and a greater openness of heart. . .Not only could this be the next step for humanity; it could be the next step for the evolution of life on Earth. It is possible that all of our development so far is simply paving the way for this inner exploration—the exploration not just of the mind, but of consciousness itself.

If this is so, then Robert Monroe, pioneer of exploration into consciousness, has shown humanity a way to take that step.

The Monroe System

TAPES

Most of the tapes referred to in these chapters come from four different series. Each tape carries appropriate phased sound signals.

Gateway Experience

This is an in-home training system comprising six volumes of taped exercises, each containing six tapes. Tapes from volumes 1-4 are among those used in the Gateway Voyage residential program.

Volume 1, *Discovery*, introduces tools, exercises, and experiences that help the listener to relax, attune to the process, control his or her own energy, handle and dispose of anxieties and worries, and explore the "world" of Focus 10. Tape 2, *Introduction to Focus 10*, which incorporates a detailed physical and mental relaxation process, is often used as an adjunct to therapeutic treatment.

Volume 2, *Threshold,* moves into Focus 12 and deals with problem-solving and patterning—a technique for enabling one to take charge of one's own life—and includes exercises for directing energy, working with colors to activate your own energy (Tape 4, *Color Breathing*), and balancing and strengthening the physical body (Tape 6, *Living Body Map*). Most exercises used in professional and practical work come from Volumes 1 and 2.

Volumes 3, *Freedom,* and 4, *Adventure,* contain a variety of exercises and experiences in Focus 10 and 12; volumes 5 and 6 (*Exploring* and *Prospecting*) consist of musical compositions with Hemi-Sync signals for individual practice and exploration.

Mind Food

Most of the tapes in this series are for practical application in everyday situations, while others offer techniques and experiences for personal development. For a full list see Addenda.

Metamusic

These are musical compositions incorporating Hemi-Sync signals which provide mental and physical relaxation and offer opportunities for heightened creativity and reduction of stress. They are also widely used as background to treatment; for example, they can be effective in dentistry, massage, psychotherapy, and therapeutic work with children.

Inner Journey, Sleeping Through the Rain, Midsummer Night, and *Sunset* are among the Metamusic tapes referred to in the text.

Human Plus (H-PLUS)

This series consists of more than fifty taped exercises designed to help one establish control over one's total self, in order to enhance and improve all factors in daily life. It is described as "a system of planned self-evolution."

Each tape teaches the listener to open and use an Access Channel, which transmits communication to all levels of awareness—physical, mental, and emotional. With the Access Channel open, a specific brain/body state is anchored to a short verbal cue or Function Command. The desired state may then be re-created at will simply by using the Function Command during daily activities.

In effect, H-PLUS is a learning system, requiring the active participation of the listener. The learning is cumulative; the system's efficiency increases with the more Functions that are learned and the frequency with which they are used. Functions may be combined to suit specific needs. While some Functions become more effective over time with regular use, others become operational almost immediately. In some instances, the Function Command becomes permanently installed at the first hearing of the tape; most of these are directed toward general well-being through enhancement of physical health and balance.

There is no restriction on the use of H-PLUS other than that imposed by one's own belief system. If you believe that you *cannot* do something, you are very unlikely ever to be able to do it. The belief, or better still the knowledge, that you can do something strengthens your ability to do it. Substitution of a *know* system for a belief system enables you to achieve extra-ordinary performance and to surpass what you formerly assumed to be your limitations. A complete list of the H-PLUS exercises may be found in the Addenda.

Explorer Tapes

These are recordings made during laboratory sessions with subjects using Hemi-Sync to achieve altered states of consciousness.

Time Out for Sleep

A programmable compact disc enabling you to set your own pattern of sleep.

Emergency Series

A set of six tapes for use principally before, during, and after surgery.

Stroke Recovery

A set of six tapes designed to aid recovery from the effects of a stroke by helping to renew the speech centers, restore motor response, and improve mental and emotional states.

RESIDENTIAL COURSES

The Monroe Institute offers four different residential courses: Gateway Voyage, Guidelines, Lifeline, and Life Span 2000.

Gateway Voyage

The Gateway Voyage program consists of a series of prerecorded exercises utilizing the frequency following response, Hemi-Sync, and vocal guidance to achieve progressive states of consciousness. These exercises are heard through stereo headphones while in a relaxed position in an individual-controlled holistic environment unit (known as a CHEC unit), under the supervision of experienced trainers. Reinforcement in learning such states is enhanced by lectures, discussions, and individual interviews. The six-day program is open to individuals who are intellectually curious or possess latent talents and abilities, subject to acceptance by the program review board.

Guidelines

Guidelines is a "graduate" program for those who have participated in the Voyage. It builds on the tools already mastered and the experiences achieved and offers advanced training in Focus 15 and 21. The participant learns to move into states of awareness in which contact with an "inner self helper" may be made, and to report on communication received. The program also gives direct training in the early stages of out-of-body work. A personal session in the laboratory isolation booth is included.

Lifeline

Lifeline is also a "graduate" program. It has the theme of service to others, particularly those no longer in time-space physical existence. It is the most powerful learning experience the Institute has so far attempted, with participants operating in Focus levels 22-27.

Life Span 2000

Life Span 2000 is an intense learning system, developed from the Human Plus series of exercises, aimed at providing means and methods for living progressively and constructively in a rapidly changing world environment. Hence it helps participants to master all the functions and abilities in the full H-PLUS list (see Addenda), with the addition of new functional learning patterns to supply other potentials that may be needed.

Full details of all courses are obtainable from The Monroe Institute, Rt 1, Box 175, Faber, VA 22938-9749; telephone 804-361-1500 or 1252.

Details of Outreach weekend courses and other workshops may also be obtained from the Institute.

The Monroe Institute encourages the use of its products by other organizations while ensuring that such use is appropriate and in accordance with its own aims and purposes. The term Hemi-Sync is a registered trade mark of the Institute. If in doubt as to whether the use of the technology and/or the terminology by another organization or individual has been authorized, please contact the Institute.

Applications: Body

Chapter 1
The Challenge of Surgery

The Emergency Series is a set of six tapes created to provide help through physical crises such as major illness, traumatic injury, or surgery. The exercises are planned to reinforce the ability of the mind to enhance the physical, mental, and emotional components of the total healing process. The mind is encouraged to direct the autonomic body functions to accelerate healing while reducing pain and discomfort. At the same time, the listener is helped to achieve and maintain a relaxed, confident, and positive attitude.

Each tape carries specific sound signals, designed to bring about an internal environment of calm and relaxation and to lead the listener into focused states of consciousness productive for recovery from illness or injury. Tapes 1 through 5 carry appropriate verbal instructions and encodings to guide the listener through the process and to help with alleviating tension and reducing the perception of pain.

Tape 1: *Pre-Op.* This exercise, for use preceding surgery, following injury, or for general health maintenance, guides the listener into deep relaxation and sleep.

Tape 2: *Intra-Op.* This is for use immediately prior to and during surgery (if this is practicable). The patient is led through processes of balancing the total system, experiencing serenity, and perceiving an absence of pain.

Tape 3: *Recovery.* The guidance given in Tape 2 is continued and the patient is led gently into wakefulness. This exercise may be used in the Recovery Room.

Tape 4: *Recuperation* or *Pain Control.* This is an exercise which helps the listener to sleep and also to reduce the perception

27

of pain. It may be used in Intensive Care, in the hospital ward, or at any time to reduce anxiety or pain and promote sleep.

Tape 5: *Energy Walk*. This guided visualization supports the healing process and is designed to restore and balance the listener's energy and establish a feeling of well-being.

Tape 6: *Surf*. This is a tape carrying no verbal instructions, consisting of sound signals embedded in the soothing rhythms of ocean waves and establishing an environment conducive to deep relaxation.

With reference to Tapes 2 and 3, recent studies have demonstrated that patients who are completely anesthetized may still register much of what is happening around them. Indeed, they may understand enough of what is said during surgery to affect the course of recovery (see *Anesthesiology*, September 1989, and *The Lancet*, August 1988). At a symposium on Memory and Awareness in Anesthesia, held at Glasgow University in 1989, Dr. Henry Bennett, of the University of California Medical School at Davis, said, "Studies show that language understanding continues during anesthesia, though explicit recall of what is said does not. But the understanding is enough to allow patients to recognize meanings of what is said and to respond later without consciously remembering what was said to them."

In some hospitals the surgeon or anesthesiologist may introduce the patient to the Emergency Series. "Over the years we have used the Emergency Series for many types of surgical procedures with great success," said Dr. Arthur Gladman, of Oakland, California, who used the tapes himself when he underwent surgery. Dr. Peter Kozicky, an orthopedic surgeon at St. Luke's Hospital in Bethlehem, noted that patients who had used the tapes for major surgery found a significant reduction in pain experienced afterwards and also in "that constant psychological turmoil that people go through." However, it is more usual for the patient to bring the tapes into the hospital and seek permission from the professionals to be allowed to use them.

This chapter begins with Gari Carter's description of her experiences stretching over ten years following a near-fatal car accident, adapted from her forthcoming book *Healing Myself*. Next, Mary Lou Ballweg, co-founder of the Endometriosis Association, explains why her fifth operation was so different from the preceding four. Lastly, Dr. Robert Roalfe, until recently a senior anesthesiologist in Oakland, California, provides an account of his use of the Emergency Series with hospital patients.

As this volume goes to press, clinical trials of the Emergency Series involving the experiences of several hundred patients are in progress.

Healing Myself
Gari Carter

In February 1982, Gari Carter and her eleven-year-old son Tom were driving along a narrow country road in Virginia. They were on their way to Baltimore to select spring items for her clothing and gift shop. It was snowing and the road was icy. They debated about whether to continue and decided to give it another five minutes to see if conditions might change. The five minutes were nearly up when a station wagon appeared around a curve, lost control, and headed straight for them. There was neither space nor time to pull off the road. Gari's one thought was for the safety of her son; she pulled sharply to the left, but her car lacked power to make it into the other lane in time. The station wagon hit them head-on.

Miraculously, Tom was uninjured. A cloth trash bag had flown into his face, protecting him from broken glass. But Gari's face was crushed between the steering wheel and the headrest, and the engine was jammed into her legs, nearly severing her right leg and breaking almost every bone between her hips and her toes.

Tom got out and tried to help Gari, but discovered she was not breathing. Using his Boy Scout CPR training—and how he did it when her face was "one big open gory hole" Gari never knew—he managed to help her start to breathe again. But there was no way he could drag her out of the wrecked car. A woman living in a trailer nearby was letting her cat out at the time; she saw and heard the crash, sent her husband to do what he could, and phoned for help. A passing driver stopped, extinguished flames he saw flickering under the hood, and stayed with Gari until the first Rescue Squad arrived. The Squad had only recently been able to afford a "Jaws of Life" machine, which tore the car apart so that she could be freed. Gari and Tom were taken to the University of Virginia Hospital in Charlottesville, while another squad took the four students in the station wagon to the Fredericksburg Hospital.

As it happened, the UVA Hospital was one of only five in the U.S.A. at that time which had a Craniofacial Clinic in its Plastic

Surgery Department, where doctors work on the underlying bones as well as the face in reconstruction. On her arrival, both Craniofacial Plastic Surgeons and Orthopedists quickly began work.
The story of what followed is told in Gari's own words, adapted from her forthcoming book Healing Myself.

First a tracheotomy incision was made into my throat and a tracheostomy tube inserted so that my breathing could be controlled and the doctors could manage anesthesia without my having a nose or mouth. Next the orthopedic surgeons repaired my almost-severed leg, reattaching all the numerous minute muscles, nerves, and ligaments and salvaging what they could of my shattered patella. They set the broken bones and put gauze dressings and splints on them. The leg lacerations were sutured to heal before putting on casts at a later date.

Meanwhile, the plastic surgeons were stitching the layers of my face back together. As the hole reached from my neck to my eyes, they began at the deepest part under the eyes, working down and out. I later learned to my frustration that repairing a face is like constructing a house. You have to have a firm foundation inside before you can start on what is seen outside. At this point, the important thing was to close up all wounds as fast as possible so that I would survive. Later they would be able to operate to repair and restructure the bones. By then I had lost a good deal of blood, and there was concern about saving my life. I had never broken any bones before, or been hurt in any way, so had no idea of what I was to go through in the next nine years. . .

I have fleeting impressions of my time in limbo. When one is in a coma, the sense of hearing is sometimes still there. I could not talk, as the tracheostomy controlled my shallow breathing; moreover, my face was sewn up to heal. I could not taste anything without a mouth to eat—all my nourishment came from intravenous feeding. I could not smell without a nose. I could touch only with my right hand as all the rest of my body was either tied or weighted down. I did not want to move owing to the incredible stabs of pain. There was a huge totality of pain in every particle of my body. I simply existed inside my pain-filled shell. It was like a symphony: suddenly different unimaginable spots would be featured, catching me off guard with new pain which overrode the background hurts. My existence flowed, pain without ceasing. I had no idea where I was or what had happened to me. I was in a new, unknown, incongruous world populated with strangers, in which I had lost all former memory of

31

who I'd been. I did not know where I lived. Did I have a family? I really did not care. I just wanted the intense, enveloping pain to stop.

When I floated into semi-alertness, I would hear flashes of loud conversations in foreign medical language and not understand how they related to me. Some people would talk as if I were not able to hear them. Others talked as if I could answer, though there was no chance. Some had gentle, soft touches and were thoughtful in the way they did whatever they had to do with me. Others jerked and pummelled me like a huge truck mashing me, immersing me with more incredible, overwhelming hurts. There were noises of bells ringing, rattling carts, wheelchairs rolling, shuffling people walking, fast purposeful people walking in squishy rubber-soled shoes—a strange assortment of noises to identify. I was attached to the real world only with my ears. I felt maimed and lost without my other senses. All these fleeting impressions did not add up: I felt as if I were in a strange prison of insistent torturing pain. I did not care enough to find out where I was or who I was or why I was there before floating back into merciful unconsciousness. . .

The plastic surgeon who would painstakingly construct my new face was Dr. Milton T. Edgerton, Chief of the Craniofacial Clinic. I felt lucky to be a patient of his. He had an outstanding medical background, ranging from his work with early pioneers in plastic surgery on soldiers after World War II in Valley Forge General Hospital to his work at Johns Hopkins Hospital and the University of Virginia Hospital, at both of which he had organized, started, and directed the Craniofacial Surgery programs. He was a real trailblazer in grafting techniques and had been a visiting professor of plastic surgery in India, Rochester, Washington, Chicago, Yale, and Toronto. I had read a book a few years earlier, *A Face for Me* by Debbie Diane Fox, concerning Dr. Edgerton's ground-breaking surgical transformation of her disfigured face, involving movement of her eyes from the sides to the front of her face and construction of fingers from her toes. I never dreamed I would be needing his expertise in a similar way, but here I was and grateful to have such a qualified surgeon.

Dr. Edgerton introduced me to Dr. Robert Chuong, who had a similar gentle touch. They examined my face meticulously. Their plans were to refracture my jaws to make them fit, reconstruct my cheeks, start shaping lips, and smooth lumps from the broken bones around my eyes where possible. This would all be internal work, so the outside would not change yet. I found it incredibly frustrating to have to wait for the foundation to be built when all I wanted was the

32

outer appearance. In the future a nose would be made for me, teeth fitted into my new jaws, then lips grafted and shaped in several steps. Each time, the scars would be reduced as much as possible. I could not help feeling hopeful for the future after listening to their careful plans.

Further surgery followed a few months later, including bone grafts to reconstruct upper and lower jaws and cheekbones, skin grafts for gum tissue, and construction of teeth. Surgeries were spaced about six months apart to allow for adequate healing, which was interminable, painful, and unendurable. I was able to have only liquids with a Brecht feeder (a syringe with a rubber tube), so nutrition and vitamins were minimal. Memory loss was intensified by each anesthesia and codeine use, delaying my recovery. . .

As time passed, I longed for my former independence. It was a long, laborious process of becoming my second self, inside and out. I not only had to relearn physical and mental abilities in new ways in order to survive, but also had to craft and shape the new person I was to be. My first personality was constantly remolded by what the people around me wanted me to be. I used to change like a chameleon if I felt I was not fitting in. Now I was physically prevented from performing my old roles. I was forced to watch life go by me and be quiet. I was able to think how I felt about other people's behavior and morals, and I could finally decide what I would and would not accept. With my second chance at life, I determined to hold fast to my own beliefs and ideals. I kept true to loving others as I wished to be loved and found myself showered with wonderful people and events. I no longer worried about making others' lives perfect for them. Facing my own recovery consumed all my thoughts and time. I realized it was better to show others the way to help themselves and not to do it all for them. I would never again take for granted all the abilities as I did in my first life. Each was too hard-won this time.

A magical event was to make my outlook very positive before my next surgery, despite my fears of the pain and trauma to come. A friend called to tell me of some surgery pain-control tapes she had heard about which helped one to recover faster. If she had not been insistent I would never have pursued the matter; so many well-meaning friends had suggested things to help me and I had learned to thank them for their concern and do as I wished afterwards. Anyway, I phoned the Monroe Institute and Helen Warring, the Registrar, said that the Emergency Series would be perfect for my needs with future surgery. She described the hemispheric synchronization process, which transports the listener into specific expanded states of consciousness, in my case to assist me to heal rapidly and ignore pain. It sounded like a magic door opening into freedom from pain.

The next surgery involved removing a rib to shape and insert as a nose, refracturing and resetting the bones in the orbits around my eyes, and repairing my sinuses. I was terrified at the prospect of renewed pain and was unwilling to trust the Emergency Series, despite the recommendation. Anyway, I listened to all the tapes when they arrived and then used the *Pre-Op* exercise twice daily in the week before surgery was due. My body calmed itself in places where I had not realized I was tense. Robert Monroe's calm voice guided me through a total body relaxation into sleep. A code is given to help you relax: "From this moment on, whenever you desire to relax and remove all harmful tension and emotion from your mind and body, all you need do is think of the number ten, inhale deeply, and exhale as if you are blowing out a candle." To have this secret ten code made me feel powerful and free.

Dr. Edgerton was happy to allow me to use the tapes, and a student nurse was assigned to observe and report on their effect. My mother had made a sign that was fixed above my bed: "Pain control tapes in use—please do not touch or talk to patient." The nurse took my blood pressure and temperature before administering any medication and was amazed at how they were lowered after I listened to the *Pre-Op* tape. I was given my preliminary medication and waited. . .and waited. I was relaxed but not bored, listening to my *Pre-Op* tape over and over. Finally the nurse returned and told me there had been an emergency surgery so mine was to be delayed by several hours. I was relieved that the bed next to mine was empty, affording me privacy and quiet to immerse myself in Hemi-Sync tranquility. I reflected on my former anxiety and was grateful for the gift of this calm oasis.

Eventually the orderly arrived for me. I switched tapes to *Intra-Op*, and as I slid on to the operating table I felt warm and secure and in control of myself at long last. After Dr. Edgerton discussed with me the shape of nose I would prefer, the anesthesiologist asked if I was ready to start. I reminded him to make sure my tapes were ready for me in the recovery room and said he could begin.

The *Intra-Op* tape repeats, in Robert Monroe's calm, trustworthy voice, "You are not alone," over and over. Hearing this made me feel totally supported by the surgical team and the entire world. The surgery lasted four and a half hours as they removed my designated rib, closed up that incision, refractured and repaired my sinus cavities, refractured and straightened the bones in the orbits around my eyes, carved and inserted the rib to make my nose, pulled skin from the sides of the face to cover it, and then finally reconstructed nostrils.

I spent the rest of the day resting and listening to *Recovery,* the *Energy Walk* visualization, and the *Pain Control* tape whenever I felt a twinge of pain. The code for pain control is "When you consciously wish to turn down [pain signals from your physical body] until they are no longer important, all you need do is, first, look with your closed eyes at that part of your physical body which is the source of such signals; second, as you look, repeat in your mind the number 55515." It worked! I never needed any pain medication after the surgery, which relieved the nurses of paying me extra attention. They were both glad and amazed that my experiment was working. Dr. Edgerton was impressed that I had a minimal amount of swelling and no black eyes or bruising and healed so quickly on my own, so much so that next morning my IVs were removed—previously I had to continue on them for several days, imprisoning me and depressing me further. I felt hopeful that I could conquer the world with these tapes now. It was such a gift to control my own pain when I needed and not be at the mercy every three hours of a codeine shot. I felt I had graduated from victim status into harmonious control.

I persuaded my doctors to let me use the Emergency Series in the operating room from then on. The next two surgeries were to attach Abbe flaps from my palate to the future lip area, allowing the grafted flaps to heal in place, and to sculpt lips from the joined tissue. Dr. Edgerton was interested to see what effect the tapes would have on me during surgery. The wires from the earbud speakers would have to be wound under my neck and attached to the tape player above my head to ensure sterility, and a nurse would be assigned to flip tapes each forty-five minutes as they ended.

I was calm the night before in the hospital listening to *Pre-Op* and was glad the sign above my bed—"Do not touch or talk to patient when using pain control tapes"—was in place. I was tranquilly grateful for the Monroe tapes after visiting hours were over. Instead of my old feelings of isolation, terror, and queasiness in my solar plexus and an urgency to get up and run out of the hospital so I would not have to go through all the hurt next day, I was calmed and soothed by Robert Monroe's voice telling me to relax. I fell asleep listening to the *Pre-Op* tape. When I awoke I used *Pain Control* to remind myself of the codes to relax and delete pain signals. It was easier this time since I knew what to expect.

It was a relief not to shake the stretcher with fear on my ride to the operating room. The trip was swift and pleasant while I listened to my *Intra-Op* tape. The nurse putting in the IV needle asked about the tapes. All the medical personnel seemed interested in the principle, and it seemed strange to me that this process was not more widely used. They arranged my tape player on the operating table above my head and threaded the wires from the earphones under my neck and up the left side of my head.

Dr. Edgerton reminded me that he would use Xylocaine locally and that I was not to move my face or mouth while he worked. He would leave a small opening on the side for me to eat with Brecht feeders during the weeks of graft healing. I drifted off with *Intra-Op* and Robert Monroe's voice telling me that I was not alone and everyone was there to help me. I knew I was in the best possible hands. I could feel a slight pulling and cutting of my face at times, but no pain.

Suddenly the absence of the tape sound jarred me alert. I opened my eyes and saw Dr. Edgerton's face directly over mine as he concentrated on his work. I remembered that I was not to move my face and tried blinking to get his attention, but without success. Then I tried rolling my eyes toward the tape player above my head to make him realize it had stopped. Surely the nurse assigned to it would notice! I felt a panicky scream rising in my throat while I tried frantically to think of what else I could do to get their attention. Finally I realized I could make a noise without moving my mouth and said "Mmmm, mmmm, mmmm." Dr. Edgerton looked startled, not expecting his patient to talk to him on the table. I rolled my eyes toward the tape player and the nurse checked it. My batteries had run out! "I only have a little more to do on your chin," said Dr. Edgerton. "Can you hold on for me?" I started to nod my head but caught myself in time and murmured "mmm hmm," hoping he would understand. I was trapped and had no choice. He had been his usual kind self, thinking of my feelings, though he wanted to finish just like any artist.

I had to try to re-create the tape by myself as he finished the surgery. I did not allow myself to slip away into the cold sterile terror of the operating room. I visualized my face with closed eyes. I told the pain signals to go away with 55515. I resolved to remember that I had done this before. I would overcome the latest obstacles and clutch my shreds of calm tightly to my inner self. I amazed myself by faintly savoring that relaxing peace with each careful breath.

As he finished, Dr. Edgerton patted my shoulder. "You were

terrific, Gari. Do you have extra batteries?" To my great relief new batteries were brought to me in the recovery room. I would never go into the operating room again without new batteries and backups! I switched on the *Pain Control* tape and blissfully slept. Later I found out that the surgery had lasted five hours, longer than anticipated, hence the batteries' demise.

Two Abbe flaps had been used, instead of one as planned, to obtain enough vermilion for lips from the area left inside the palate. One month of healing was needed before the next surgery to sever and sculpt the graft. The rest of my cheeks and chin were a road map of suture lines. I could neither talk, smile, nor spit and would be unable to vomit. Every operation seemed to bring new adjustments which I never thought about in advance. I used the *Energy Walk* exercise and positive visualizations for healing. I wanted to heal quickly so that I could talk and eat again. . .

In a month I returned to UVA for lip sculpture, chin and cheek shaping, and tracheotomy revision, with brand-new batteries for my tape player. I relished my confident calmness as surgery seemed to flash by. My chin was slowly taking shape to look real, the cheeks were less sunken, I had lips, and the big, jagged tracheotomy scar was a thin line. Dr. Edgerton found and removed an adhesion the size of a little finger which had grown around my vocal cords and had caused me pain when swallowing. I healed rapidly and uneventfully, enjoying my new freedom. When the final sutures were out, I had to learn how to aim a fork into my new, narrow mouth and guide a glass to my mouth with my tongue instead of my senseless lips. . .

By the next surgery my tapes were accepted by the nurses and doctors as a part of me. In the hospital the night beforehand, however, I lay in bed overwhelmed by anguish and loneliness. I missed my mother, who was usually with me, and wondered if I would be strong enough to survive yet another surgery the next day. I longed for someone to give me a compassionate hug to erase my forlornness. Tears of self-pity streaked down my cheeks. I stared, without seeing, at the ugly green hospital chair and trite painting of a field and a pond. As I wallowed in my despair, the room slowly changed. The chair gave off a glowing aura, as did the painting, the foot of the bed, and even the silent television impaled high on the wall. They all exuded a lovely embracing happiness with me, like a shiny Christmas tree. I understood in a flash of peace in my heart that all these ugly things were there to help me heal, just like the doctors and nurses. I realized that I should never feel alone again. We are constantly surrounded by love and healing wherever we are. The green chair was teaching me just what I tried to teach others about myself. Inside an ugly exterior beams a true shining light. The whole sweep of my journey to find myself was resolved in that instant, and I whispered "Thank you" to the glowing green chair and the rest of the room. I turned on my tape player to ready myself for the battle of surgery the next day.

This five-hour surgery included more grafting to even the lips and prevent drooling, Z-plasties in chin scars, sculpting an indentation below my lips to separate the chin, and revision of knee scars. . . .Later, I was nervous about pain from the removal of the pull lines on my knee but repeated "55515" while I visualized the area with closed eyes, as I had been told to do on the tape, and erased all pain signals. . .

The next-to-last surgery involved more Z-plasties in the chin, resculpting the indentation under the lips, additional reshaping of the lips to prevent drooling, removal of a growth on my foot at the point of a broken bone, and removal of cysts on suture lines on my upper eyelids. The confusion of getting ready for the operating room washed over me without effect due to the strong inner calm from the *Pre-Op* tape. This surgery seemed to last a fraction of a minute although I later found it had been another five hours.

In the recovery room I listened to just one side of the *Recovery* tape and then felt ready to return to my own room, where I relaxed into *Energy Walk*, noticing that I now had a roommate. At midnight the lady yelled, "Ethel, get my shoes!" I thought she was dreaming and turned on my tape player. I was almost asleep when she yelled again. I told her Ethel was not there and shoes were not needed in bed. She kept yelling, so I rang for the nurse, who explained that she was senile. One needs quiet to use the tapes properly, and I was unable to keep my calm, pain-free state with the unexpected interruptions and had to ask for codeine. The next day, I felt drugged, dizzy, and weak. It made me realize that my body did not want to take drugs anymore. I was much better off with the tapes, if I had the privacy to use them. . .

After the lips were finished, I began speech therapy—a major challenge without feeling in my grafted lips. Since I was told to relax before I began, I used my Emergency Series tapes and then practiced smiling, swallowing, and rounding my lips as I watched in a mirror. I had to practice my speech laboriously on tape, exercising my weak lip and cheek muscles. Most difficult was re-learning how to laugh. Slowly I could hear progress, but my voice would never regain the strength, range, or volume it had before, as only one vocal cord would work properly. At least it was low and pleasing to the ear. . .

The final surgery in October 1990 was filmed by The Monroe Institute. We began with a short interview in which I described my introduction to the tapes. We toured the Virginia Ambulatory Surgery Center and then moved to the waiting room. Here the television was blaring full blast and a baby was throwing noisy toys and crying in the play area while his mother watched impassively. I despaired of finding my peace and solitude in this miasma of agitation. I sat as far from the noise as possible, put on my earphones, and turned the volume up as high as possible. I called on every shred of concentration in my being to block out the waiting room din. Thanks again to Robert Monroe's calm, reassuring voice, I succeeded. I was startled away from my inner self by hearing my name called and opened my eyes to see that I was being filmed. The nurse had called me into the preparation area. As I followed her, I felt grateful to be walking into surgery this time instead of being pushed on a stretcher. My current well-being was invaluable to me now!

Dr. Edgerton surprised me as I concentrated on my tapes. We discussed the forthcoming surgery and he told me we were both to give interviews to the film crew before the operation took place. During the interview I said how much I appreciated that Dr. Edgerton allowed me to use the tapes and to be filmed during an operation. This filming might help to open other people's eyes to being pain-free. I also mentioned a recent visit I had made to the Institute and the developments I had seen there, including the installation of a NRS-24 Neuromapper and the launching of the Human Plus tape series.

As Dr. Edgerton began working on my face I felt an uncontrollable butterfly of tension emerge in my solar plexus. I doubted my stamina and concentration abilities and realized I needed more help. I did not want to break down in front of the camera and ruin the film, after all the help the Institute had given me.

I asked, "Could I please have something to take off the edge?" I did not say "edge of terror" but meant it. Dr. Edgerton ordered a small dose of Demerol. I realized that I deserved the extra sedation as Dr. Edgerton's surgeries were legendary in length owing to his meticulous art.

I felt myself flying down the sliding board of oblivion with the Demerol and was able to concentrate on my tape as the tension flew up and out of me. When I really concentrate in the operating room, I feel totally disassociated from my body as if I were on the ceiling dispassionately observing what the surgeons are doing. My body registers pricks from Xylocaine and pushing, cutting, and stitching without a care or any reaction, while my spirit floats in happiness. I can only liken it to the exhilaration of skiing when one feels as if one were flying or sailing when the wind is just right and one skims the water. I always experience great resistance leaving that state of perfect bliss.

Dr. Edgerton made a W-plasty to a grooved scar in the chin and a Z-plasty to lengthen the left lower lip and prevent drooling, debulked the trapdoor flap in the right center anterior chin, made bilateral Z-plasties in the transverse scars running from the lower lip toward the ear regions, and excised the redundant scar tissue in the anterior lower lip. The nurse flipped my tape each time it ended, so I had continuous sound. After two hours Dr. Edgerton said he was late for his rounds and dashed off. His resident closed the last incisions and tidied me up. He asked if I wanted any pain medication.

"No thanks, the tapes are all I need," I replied through my heavy bandaging.

Filming continued as I was moved into the recovery room. I was anxious to change the *Intra-Op* tape for the *Recovery* one. My body dissolved into tiredness, though my mind was alert. They asked me if I remembered asking to have my tapes flipped during surgery.

"I most definitely remember," I said. "When the tape ends, one plummets to reality from that fluffy cloud of serenity. I felt like an addict needing a fix because I wanted that tape back on urgently without delay. When I listen to the tapes, I float above all the surgical action and am aware of what is going on from a remote perspective."

I was grateful when the camera stopped as I needed to be flat, listening to the recovery tape. I floated on my tape-induced cloud of peace, which dissolved partially and then reformed as the nurses checked on my blood pressure. I did not want the peaceful journey of recovery to end. . .

This last healing has been the best of all. I had not only the Emergency series, but the luxury of the extra back-up of the H-PLUS series to enrich my recovery. I found less need to listen to the *Pain Control* tape if I went to sleep with H-PLUS *Restorative Sleep*. I alternated H-PLUS *Regenerate, Circulation, Tune-Up* and *Emergency: Injury.* I used neuromuscular and craniosacral therapies to reduce scar tissue and rebalance my body. I felt strengthened and invigorated by so much healing help from which to choose.

My sweeping journey from independence to dependence and back filled almost ten years of my life. I now realize that my new expanded life was entwined with giving and receiving openly with those surrounding me. My life has been enriched by all those who helped me on the way to recovery. At first I longed for one mentor to sponsor me in my battle to come back after my tragedy. Since I never found my hero, I became my own, as I managed alone. I worked on mastering my goal to become a person of integrity, courage, resilience, and perseverance. My self-image was balanced now, instead of being based on outward appearances as it was in my first life. I realize that in all our lives we either experience, or have someone we love go through, difficult times in one way or another. The perception, rather than the actual incident, is of crucial importance to one's well-being. My tragedy evolved from the worst to the best event in my life. My recovery shows that the mind, body and soul can be transformed.

In his foreword to Healing Myself, *Robert Monroe describes Gari Carter's story as "fresh testimony as to the strength of the human spirit that can bring hope to those in the midst of tragedy." These extracts give some idea of the outstanding courage with which Gari confronted her experiences and of her faith and trust in herself, her doctors and, latterly, in the tapes which helped her to handle the anxiety and pain accompanying the surgery and to accelerate the healing process.*

Coping With Surgery

Mary Lou Ballweg

In 1978 Mary Lou Ballweg was diagnosed with endometriosis. This is a frequently misdiagnosed and misunderstood disease process in which tissue normally lining the uterus is also found in the abdomen and on the ovaries, bowel, and bladder. The resulting internal bleeding, scar tissue, and inflammation produce a number of debilitating symptoms including, but not limited to, chronic pelvic pain and painful menstrual periods, painful intercourse, infertility, bowel and bladder problems, chronic fatigue, and low resistance to infections. The cause is unknown and no cure is available. Treatment options include a spectrum of pain medications and a variety of traditional surgeries and new laser techniques to remove the growths. However, these frequently recur, necessitating repeated operations or hysterectomy as a last resource. Endometriosis affects an estimated five million women in the United States and another half million in Canada, with sufferers ranging from eleven to fifty years of age. In 1980, Mary Lou, together with Carolyn Keith, founded the Endometriosis Association, which offers support and assistance to those directly affected, educates the public and medical community, and promotes research related to the condition.

In the following contribution (reprinted with permission from The Endometriosis Association Newsletter, *Vol. 12, No. 6), Mary Lou describes her use of the Emergency Series to decrease pain and anxiety in recent surgical treatment.*

Facing surgery is hard! Fortunately, there's a new development in this area that can make a major difference.

It's hard to put into words the anxiety that occurs for most of us when facing surgery, even when we're well-prepared and feel confident in our surgeon. It seems that every day before surgery a certain anxious gloom pervades the mind at least part of the time, and grows in the days before the procedure. Last year when I was facing surgery again (my fifth for endometriosis) I was fortunate to find an aid that made this surgery far more emotionally manageable than my earlier ones.

At the American Association of Gynecologic Laparoscopists' annual meeting in November 1990, Dr. Ronald Burke of the University of Massachusetts Medical School presented the results of a study on which he had worked with Suzanne Jonas, Ed.D., and the Fertility Institute of Western Massachusetts, using special relaxation audio tapes. In the study, one group of patients used the tapes before coming to the hospital, while under anesthesia, and in the recovery room; a second group did not use the tapes at all. Both groups underwent diagnostic or operative laparoscopy. Dr. Burke reported that the group using the tapes had significantly less pain and nausea following their operations and returned to full activity more quickly than the control group.

Another study, reported in *The Lancet* (August 27, 1988, Vol. 2, No. 8609, p. 491) found that patients who listened to a relaxation tape during hysterectomy recovered more quickly with less fever and significantly fewer gastro-intestinal problems than patients who had been played a blank tape. Other studies have suggested that operating room sounds may be registered in the brain even though the patient is under general anesthesia, and that these sounds may influence the pace of recovery.

Part of the effect of the tapes, therefore, may be that, besides putting positive, affirming, reassuring thoughts in the patient's head, they block out operating room sounds and statements that could be disturbing. As a result of these studies, some anesthesiologists now make gentle suggestions to patients such as saying that the operation is over and a complete success and they will be waking soon and will do well.

I decided to try out the tapes used in the Jonas/Burke study for my surgery last year and to share the experiences with our members, who face so many operative laparoscopies. My general practitioner supported me in this.

I contacted The Monroe Institute and was sent the set of six tapes, the Emergency Series. As well as the audio signals, the tapes carry a very soothing voice which encourages the listener to relax. Tape one, *Pre-Op*, for instance, is a wonderfully relaxing, affirming tape in which the narrator takes the listener step by step through conscious relaxation, head to toe. *"First, let your jaw, let your jaw go limp and relax, let the muscles and nerves of your jaw go limp and relax. Now, your eyelids. Let your eyelids relax and go limp. Now, let your lips, let the muscles and nerves in your lips relax, relax easily and go limp. Now, the muscles in your forehead. . . "* Chances are that by the end of the tape you're asleep, or at the least very relaxed and no longer anxious.

The instructions note that you should use the *Pre-Op* tape as many times as possible prior to surgery, before and after admission to hospital. I found this tape unbelievably soothing and used it several times before surgery. One night I found it hard to sleep—I was anxious and the persistent, intermittent sound of the foghorn out on Lake Michigan bothered me. I hoped the tape would knock out the foghorn sound; although it didn't, it made me feel so good and relaxed that I wasn't bothered by the foghorn any more. After the surgery I realized that the tape did the same thing with pain and discomfort; it was still there but didn't bother me, just as the tape said.

It was suggested to me that I kept notes on my use of the tapes. Here are some of the comments I wrote at the time:

Several times anxiety hits me and I listen to the *Pre-Op* or *Intra-Op* and find, despite my thoughts still being somewhat anxious, that I'm surprisingly calm and feel an inner peace. After a disconcerting doctor visit and as anxiety builds the night before, the tapes help.

The morning of the surgery I listened to them at 5:15 A.M. on the way to the hospital. I listened waiting to be taken down to surgery and in the pre-op area. I discussed them with the anesthesiologist; he's very interested and more than willing to help by being sure the earphones stay on during surgery and by replacing the *Intra-Op* with the *Recovery* tape when I go into the recovery room.

I woke in the recovery room to the soothing sounds of the tape. . . *Let the others help you restore your balance. . .You accept the green, blue, and purple healing energy that they are bringing to you; the bright, healing, warm energy they are giving to you. . .The nerve signals of pain flow through you and do not register during this period now. . .*

It was a far better way to wake than after my previous four surgeries when I remembered waking either to searing pain in the laparotomies or the dread feeling of not quite knowing where I was and being in a haze. The tape made me feel that, although

I was feeling pain, I would be able to manage it, and I was! It helped me feel that I could manage until my blood pressure came up a little and they could give me an injection of Demerol.

Later I learned that while I was listening to the *Intra-Op* tape during the surgery, the surgeon and anesthesiologist listened to some of the *Recovery* tape. In one place it says that the caregiver should check that the message is going into the right ear of the patient. They joked that they hadn't known they should check and wondered if it had rearranged the hemispheres in my brain. Was I left-handed now?

Tuesday, the day after surgery. On the *Recuperation* tape the soothing voice says that the pain signals are no longer important for now, to allow you to sleep. I like that very much; a way to be aware of what's happening to your body so you can take the necessary pain medication, or rest, or try not to do too much, yet at the same time not to let the pain and discomfort messages take over. It helps impart or put you in touch with a wonderful sense of equilibrium.

Wednesday, second day after surgery. I feel better but then become restless, a little blue, irritable about the music and voices upstairs—is this the third-day blues? I put the *Recuperation* tape on and despite my restlessness and inability to sleep find a sense of peace and relaxation. It's amazing how effective these tapes are. As one woman wrote about her spleen surgery: "Every sound and word took on a special therapeutic meaning."

Fifth day after surgery. So sore—I overdid it yesterday! I felt so good I forgot I wasn't really supposed to be out more than three or so hours. I feel good, though sore, just no energy. I want to read but don't have the energy, not really tired enough to sleep so sew instead while listening to the post-op tape called, appropriately, *Energy Walk*. The soothing voice guides the listener to imagine being on a beach, a grassy meadow, and looking at your favorite tree at the end of the meadow. It's really quite beautiful.

These tapes seem to be designed by people who have been through this. I didn't know this is what I would need after the *Recuperation* tape but here it is and perfect for what I need today:

You step into the grass and you feel it soft and cool under your feet. You feel the living green of the grass, the energy of the grass. The green energy is very special. You need to feel much more of this balancing energy, of the green in the grass, so you drop down and lie in the cool, green grass, lie down in the cool green grass, roll in it and feel a balancing, freshening energy in the grass, feel it move throughout your entire self...

Apart from the surgery, the tape even helped us on a trip when our nine-year-old developed bronchitis and a touch of pneumonia. Imagine being cooped up with a sick child in a motel room while awaiting surgery! She was so uncomfortable and restless she couldn't sleep, so I gave her the *Energy Walk* tape because the description suggests playing this tape whenever the person is "restless, in pain, or unable to sleep." Our daughter went from being restless, frustrated (and frustrating her parents) to lying perfectly still, eyes closed, smiling, relaxed. "This is wonderful, Mom. It's so beautiful. I feel so good." She drifted off into a light nap after a while.

We encourage chapters and support groups to obtain a set of the Emergency Series tapes for lending to members at the time of surgery. Encourage your doctor and hospital to obtain a set for loan to women due for surgery.

The Endometriosis Association has recently acquired 100 sets of the Emergency Series for the benefit of their members and support groups across the U.S.A. and Canada. The International Headquarters of the Association is at 8585 North 76th Place, Milwaukee, WI 53223; telephone 800-992-3636 in U.S.A., and 800-426-2363 in Canada.

Using Hemi-Sync With Surgical Patients

R. Roalfe, M.D.

Dr. Robert Roalfe, who recently retired from the post of senior anesthesiologist at a hospital in Oakland, California, was one of the first doctors to introduce patients to the Emergency Series. He reports here on the experience of more than eighty patients who used the series when undergoing surgery.

A discussion of the experiences of individual patients will illustrate the range of response, the range of patients, and what the system—and the patients themselves—and the surgery have allowed me to do in using the Hemi-Sync technology in addition to the traditional anesthesia.

The first patient I wish to discuss is actually the man who introduced me to Hemi-Sync in the first place, and who is himself a doctor: Dr. Arthur Gladman. I had the good fortune to be assigned to him as his anesthesiologist. I recognized his name and knew something of his reputation as someone interested and involved in new methods of healing and pain control, and I anticipated introducing him to some of my new techniques to see how he would respond.

When I called to introduce myself to him, I found Dr. Gladman sitting on his bed with earphones on. I apologized for interfering with his enjoyment of the music, and he replied that he was not listening to music but to some tapes. He explained these tapes to me and asked if I would mind his using them while he was in the operating theatre and in the recovery room afterwards. I was happy with this, and so it happened.

Dr. Gladman's operation was for spinal stenosis, a condition in which there is an overgrowth or impingement of the bone of the spinal column so that it presses on the spinal cord or the nerve, causing sensory and/or motor deficit. Once before he had undergone surgery for this problem, and one reason he was using the tapes was because he had, he said, suffered a really miserable surgical experience, which he described in great and grisly detail. He felt he had not been properly prepared beforehand; he went into the operating room anxious; although the surgery was uncomplicated, he woke up in pain in the recovery room and remembered nothing except the pain for another three or four days. Pain continued for about a week, requiring large amounts of medication. He also had a post-operative hematoma—bleeding into the wound. He left the hospital nine days after the surgery, two or three days later than would be expected after such an operation.

On this occasion he hoped to have no more medication than was absolutely necessary. I said that if he was fully relaxed he would need nothing until he entered the operating room, or just before then. This is how I act toward any patients who express concern about their bodies being poisoned with chemicals. With Dr.Gladman I gave him only a very small amount of Valium and of Pentonyl, a narcotic. These put the patient in a more receptive state so that the introduction of anesthetic is less traumatic. He remained very calm, listening to his tapes. The surgical procedure was uncomplicated and he used an incredibly small amount of anesthesia. He woke up on the way to the recovery room; he was very clear, knew exactly where he was and was still listening to his tapes. He spent about an hour and a half in the recovery room and was taken back to his ward; he had no medication in the recovery room, no medication after the surgery and left the hospital on day five.

Comparing Dr. Gladman's previous experience with this one, I felt that it justified my becoming interested in using the Hemi-Sync tapes. He provided me with a set and advised me how to use them. We discussed setting up a study to find out exactly what was going on and whether results using the tapes would be better than without their use.

So I began using this Emergency Series. To begin with, all went well and the patients were cooperative. Then I met Mary, who had been admitted early one morning for a total hip replacement that day. She was eighty-five years old and was in excellent health except for her joint disease and partial deafness. I introduced myself; she merely grunted and I felt we might not exactly hit it off—I was unlikely to reach an in-depth rapport with her. I explained what I did, but she didn't seem especially interested. I asked her if she was nervous and she said that she was, very. I asked what she was nervous about—what she was afraid of—but she could not be specific and didn't want to talk about it anyway. I handed her a little cassette player and asked if she would like to try listening to the tape which would help her relax and overcome her nervousness. "No," she said. I tried again and she said she didn't like music. I told her it was not music, just surf sounds, waves on the beach, very gentle. "I hate waves!" was the reply. They aren't really waves, I told her; just computer-generated noises, very relaxing. "I hate noise!" she said. So we agreed that she would do it her way and I would do it mine. Mary was the first—indeed the only—person so far who has outrightly rejected my offer of the tapes, although there have been a few who have refused after thinking it over.

I met George about three months after I started working with the tapes. He was forty-six years old, in middle management, and had injured his back. For several months he had tried a number of different therapies and treatments, and was eventually referred to me by a clinical psychologist who was an associate of Dr. Gladman and who, with his colleagues, had been using Monroe tapes in his own practice. He was admitted two days before his operation for x-rays to be taken, and we talked at length. He was already accustomed to the tapes, as he had been using them with the psychologist, and he began to use the *Pre-Op* tape two days before his surgery, maybe as often as twenty times. He was very relaxed when he was brought to the operating room. I gave him a fair amount of pre-operative medication, as he had been on pain medication for several weeks—and he was a big man, and I was concerned about how smooth his anesthetic course would be.

George's operation was uneventful; he required the anticipated amount of anesthetic and a lot of medication. He had an extremely painful and prolonged post-operative course and required much more pain medication than most people would. However, he used his tapes religiously; every time I saw him post-operatively he was listening to a tape—he was addicted to them. He told me they were really helping, but from a study of his chart you would have said they were useless. But in the long term he has gone back to work, he is totally pain-free, and he has gotten over all his problems. From my point of view he did not benefit from the tapes; but from his point of view they helped considerably, and I think we have to pay attention to that.

Helen and Betty came in for radical mastectomies owing to cancer of the breast. Helen was seventy-two; she had a biopsy on a Friday afternoon and next morning was called in and was told that she had cancer and was to come to the hospital on Monday morning.

She arrived at 8:00 A.M. for surgery at 10:30. As I was at work in the operating room, I did not see her until 9:30, an hour before her operation. She was sitting bolt upright; I don't think I have seen anyone more intensely anxious. She desperately wanted to put into words her distress at the prospect of losing half of what she believed was her best feature—her breast. She was an attractive, beautifully presented lady, looking about twenty years younger than her age, and she told me she was not married but she still dated. After about twenty-five minutes I had to leave to attend another patient and I asked her if she would listen to a relaxation tape. She demurred, but I asked her to try it as a favor to me, and to remove it if she didn't like it. She agreed. Ten minutes later I phoned from the operating room to see how she was and was told she was sound asleep. She had received no medication; nothing except talking to me and the tape. Her surgery was straightforward; she woke in the recovery room and needed only a minimal amount of medication. Next morning she was positively ecstatic; she dealt with everything beautifully and was fully reconciled to losing the breast—a loss which, she told me, did not change her.

Betty, aged sixty-one, was admitted under similar trying circumstances. She came in on a Friday morning about ninety minutes prior to her scheduled time for surgery. When I saw her she was sitting up in bed, looking less distraught than Helen but clearly extremely tense. One of the nurses told me that Betty had lost her son just a week ago in an accident, and that she had received her diagnosis of breast cancer only the previous day. She had no time to deal with that information. Betty told me that she felt she was in control, because if she didn't stay in control her husband would fall apart as he could not deal either with her son's death or with her cancer. Moreover, her son had been in coma for five days, during which she had sat beside him in hospital, watching him until he died. I talked to her for about forty-five minutes and finally she agreed to listen to the tapes—I think probably because she thought I wouldn't leave her alone until she did agree! Her response was almost identical to Helen's; within a few minutes she was peacefully asleep, also with no medication. These were two of the most dramatic and rewarding experiences I have had with patients.

The next patient had, for various reasons, no pre-op experience with the tapes. He was fifty-four years old and had contracted a respiratory infection. One day at work he felt unable to breathe; he was taken to an emergency room and, as he now could not breathe at all, he had an emergency intubation under great stress and difficulty while he was awake. He was diagnosed as having a very severe viral respiratory infection with inflammation of all the tissues of his upper airway. He was in the intensive care unit on a respirator for four or five days and recovered with intensive therapy and antibiotics. He left the hospital but continued to have mild breathing problems. He felt there was something in his throat; he was anxious about sleeping and about a repeat of the infection and was unhappy about the situation. Eventually he saw an ENT specialist who found there was a tumor above his vocal cords and behind his epiglottis, a very awkward place to get at. He was scheduled for a biopsy of this tumor under anesthetic, normally a very brief procedure, to be done by one of the cancer surgeons, technically very adept but inadequate as a human being. (I disliked working with him because of the way he treated his patients and the other people in the operating room. He dealt with many head and neck cases and with these patients it is difficult, if not sometimes impossible, to use tapes, and I gave up trying to do so.)

The patient was anxious about the operation and I tried to reassure him that it would be quick and there was little chance of his having to have a breathing tube inserted afterwards. But once the operation began the surgeon found it impossible to obtain a piece of tissue without the risk of causing bleeding which could not be controlled. After about an hour, while the patient's head was hyper-extended, his mouth wide open with all kinds of instruments being inserted, a lot of trauma and a lot of bleeding, it was decided to make an incision in his neck and enter the pharynx that way so the surgeon could see what he was doing. Luckily the patient's wife was in the hospital and gave her permission for this, but even so it took three hours to excise the tumor.

After about fifteen minutes in the recovery room the patient was unable to breathe. He was taken back to the operating room and a tracheotomy was performed to enable him to breathe through an opening in his neck.

Next morning I went to see him, realizing that he would be truly miserable. The whole experience had been extremely traumatic; moreover, this surgeon does not believe his patients hurt so he does not order pain medication. I obtained some and added that I would like him to try some relaxation tapes, suggesting that he might try all of them in turn. His wife agreed to oversee this.

When I returned later in the day he told me he felt a little better, but his wife said that he did not know how much better he was. The tapes sent him to sleep for about thirty minutes; then he would be in pain for a while, and then she would give him another tape, and back to sleep he would go. He continued to use tapes 4 and 5 for the next few days during his very painful process. At the end both agreed they had really helped him. This all happened without any preparation and was completely unplanned.

These cases represent a cross-section of the patients I have seen; they are good examples, though not all the cases are as dramatic. Now I would like to turn to a patient study that we undertook. For various reasons we were unable to obtain all the information we hoped for in the study design; for instance, we wished to include coronary by-pass surgery, but the cardio-vascular team would not fully cooperate. The supply of total hip-replacement patients, whom we wished to include, suddenly dried up. This also happened with mastectomy patients. We were left with patients in two categories: lumbar laminectomies and total hysterectomies. There were difficulties here too; most of the laminectomy patients were being re-operated upon and were on a much higher drug dosage as they had been in considerable pain for some time. So I felt we had to re-design the study along simpler lines. Having done that, it was possible to draw certain conclusions from the data we assembled. I had kept precise data on fifty patients in the original study, and added a further thirty-four on whom the data was not quite as comprehensive but, I felt, would be adequate. I had used the tapes with more than fifty other patients, but these had mostly been short-stay and had used some but not all of the tapes so they did not fit into a methodical study.

A simplified version of the results is as follows. I devised a rating scale from 5 to 1 to summarize the efficacy of the tapes. Of the eighty-one patients eventually included in the study, seven came into the top category—a spectacular success. Category 4 contained those patients who felt—or I felt, or we agreed—had obtained a really positive benefit from the tapes; there were thirty-one in that group. Group 3 comprised patients who said they felt the tapes helped although there was no actual evidence of this; these totalled twenty-five. Several patients in these groups wanted to buy or borrow the tapes themselves; many of them wanted their families to hear them. In group 2 we have the equivocal effects; patients who thought nothing happened, and perhaps it didn't, and patients in whom I could not detect any effect, twelve in all. In the bottom group were six patients who either refused to use the tapes or told me they did not like them and they did not help.

Summing up, it would seem that sixty-three out of eighty-one patients—77%—obtained in one way or another positive benefit from the use of the tapes. This is, I suggest, good enough to warrant further research of a controlled nature, which I hope will be carried out in the near future.

Chapter 2

Life Under Threat

A growing number of case histories reveals that by changing the patient's approach to his illness and by showing how the powers of the brain may be marshalled to direct and intensify the healing process, the hemispheric synchronization process can have a significant, sometimes dramatic, influence on the duration of illness and the speed of recovery. Several practitioners, including surgeons, physicians, psychologists, and psychotherapists, use the process with their patients and contribute to the increasing body of information through The Monroe Institute's Professional Division.

As well as making use of the Emergency Series, the doctor or therapist—or the patient—may choose from a variety of exercises, finding and using those which will suit a particular individual or a specific condition. For example, one lady with multiple sclerosis has been using ten different H-PLUS exercises for relief of symptoms, as well as Metamusic tapes; she describes H-PLUS as "an invaluable support in dealing with MS from moment to moment." Like many others, she has discovered that one advantage of Hemi-Sync is that, unlike much medication, it produces no side effects. Moreover, there are no pressures, financial or otherwise, on the practitioner or therapist to employ this method in preference to any other.

In this chapter, we look at ways in which Hemi-Sync has been, and is being, used when dealing with some serious physical conditions. Dr. Howard Schachter describes a recent study in which he used a Hemi-Sync tape to assist patients to confront their cancers and handle their own fears and responses. Rita Black, who trained with Dr. Bernie Siegel, provides an outline of her workshop for cancer patients, designed to strengthen their mental attitudes, release their fears, and fortify their bodies. There are accounts of programs for those diagnosed as HIV-positive. Next comes a summary of the use of Hemi-Sync with two patients afflicted with a condition which may be variously diagnosed as myalgic encephalomyelitis, post-viral fatigue syndrome, or Epstein-Barr syndrome. Lastly, we have two accounts of recovery from "closed-head trauma" where tapes from the H-PLUS series were employed.

In the light of these and a host of other recorded experiences, it is reasonable to assume that Hemi-Sync will have an increasingly valuable part to play in the medicine of the future.

Fear, Cancer, and Hemi-Sync:
A New Departure

Howard M. Schachter, Ph.D.

Howard Schachter is a transpersonal psychotherapist specializing in trauma and psychosocial oncology. He is a part-time professor with the University of Ottawa School of Psychology and with the Institute of Pastoral Studies, University of St. Paul, Ottawa.

In accordance with the experiential perspective on psychotherapeutic interventions, healing becomes possible when the client lives out, in the here and now, whatever "experiencing" is revealed to the therapist to be most pressing and significant. An "experiencing" is defined as "a cluster of bodily feelings, plus associated behaviors, relative to a given event." This perspective assumes that healing is a process of "wholing," or making whole, and involves the emergence of unactualized—often unconscious—personal or transpersonal material which needs to be integrated. "Wholing" is accomplished when the client is able to actualize, or "own," the emerging material as part of himself or herself in the present and is able to integrate it. The therapist's role is firstly to invite the client to live out fully that part in a form that feels good, or at least acceptable, on a physical level and secondly to enable the client to rehearse for the world outside its actualization in a socially acceptable fashion.

However, the experiential approach can often be quite terrifying as the client begins to face those feelings and behaviors which require integration. Hence many clients refuse the opportunity to begin work. Their reasons for refusing may be fear of feeling in a particular way—or of feeling anything at all, especially in an intense manner. Often, clients argue that this "feeling stuff" is silly, evincing a terror of losing or surrendering control to parts of themselves that are struggling for expression. Sometimes clients may simply refuse to look at any thing, person, or event which evokes strong, dysharmonious ("bad") feelings.

Therefore a method was needed which could help the client to relax during a session and also to lower his defenses against experiencing anything frightening or alien. It was assumed that such a method might help the client transcend the fear of those threatening parts of self (the inner potential) and foster integrative work during the session, as well as increasing the likelihood that the client would return to continue therapy.

This fear of alienated parts of oneself is especially seen when working with people who have cancer. Much fear, pain, and suffering arise when clients who are living with cancer are asked to relate to their disease. It has been found through experiential psychotherapy that clients with cancer project onto their disease the qualities of an inner, unlived experiencing that cannot or will not be integrated into their lives. This unexpressed experiencing emerges if the client is able to establish and intensify a relationship with the cancer. Not surprisingly, and owing to projection, the client then perceives and experiences the cancer as doing to him or her whatever he or she cannot live out in the external world (a dynamic known in Gestalt therapy as retroflection).

Therefore the client is encouraged to establish an explicit, feeling-based interaction or encounter with the disease in order to integrate and express the inner experience, of which the cancer is its manifestation, and in a way which promotes wellness rather than illness. From this perspective, healing involves harmonizing the relationship between the client and the cancer, with its qualities as the client perceives them. This therapeutic approach has been found to affect the cancer physiologically by bringing about a change in its oncologic status and, in some cases, remission. The role of the immune system in bringing about these effects is just beginning to be studied.

A proven method to bring about the desired relaxation effect is the use of standard relaxation techniques during hypnotherapeutic induction. However, many people are just as alienated by the use of hypnosis as they are by confronting an unintegrated experiencing. Clients have reported that both situations require surrendering control—to the therapist in hypnosis and to the unintegrated experiencing in experiential therapy. Consequently, a small pilot study of two cases was initiated to try an alternative brain/mind entrainment approach to relaxation that is relatively unobtrusive.

The Hemi-Sync process was familiar to me as a beneficial method of calming individuals while at the same time stimulating the opening of channels through which unintegrated experiential material could begin to be expressed. I decided to use this means when beginning experiential sessions with clients who evinced a fear of some inner material. The tape *Introduction to Focus 10* was selected with the clear understanding that, at the least, the client would benefit from the relaxation response fostered by listening to the tape. At all times, healing was the primary objective. For reasons given above, individuals with cancer were selected as good candidates for inclusion in the pilot study. Data were obtained from a thirty-eight-year-old male and a fifty-five-year-old female, each diagnosed with cancer, who qualified for the study because, when invited to close their eyes in their respective sessions and look at and describe their cancers, each refused to do so.

Before reporting the results, it may be helpful to clarify the premises within which the data are conceptualized. The experiential significance of a thing, person, or event is a function of the qualities it possesses. These qualities, when perceived, stimulate in the perceiver a certain response or experiencing. Therefore, the experiential significance is formally defined by whatever cluster of feelings and behaviors is lived out by the perceiver when he or she is relating to a thing, person, or event. This means that the particular meaning of the cancer depends on the individual perceiving it.

The same procedure was established with both clients. Once they had refused to encounter their cancers, it was suggested that they relax instead, and that work with respect to the cancer would be done only after listening to a tape that would likely help establish calm and relaxation. They were told to listen to the tape on a Sony Walkman with stereo headphones while sitting in a recliner, to go with whatever feelings and images the exercise might evoke, to suspend their disbelief if possible, and not to censor any feelings or images that might arise. They were to signal when the tape ended, keeping their eyes closed. At the signal, they were asked to describe their experiences with the tape and to look at, describe, and interact with their cancers.

Both clients described their experiences of the tape as creating increased calm and relaxation, although each admitted to having been somewhat apprehensive at the beginning of the exercise and attributed this anxiety to not being sure about what was going to happen. Once they had put their apprehensions and other concerns into the "Energy Conversion Box" they said they began to feel more comfortable. As the sessions continued, the calmness and relaxation deepened for both clients.

Following the sessions, both were more willing to look at their cancers than they had been previously. Images and feelings related to their cancers bubbled up reasonably easily.

The male client reported perceiving a dragon with characteristics described as unrelenting, burning (with fire), mean, and angry. He experienced a fear of being consumed (the surface, or operating, experiencing). In particular, the dragon was perceived as being able to burn him at the site on his scalp under which his tumor had been discovered.

The experiential significance of the relationship with the dragon/cancer was that its qualities stimulated the experience of being consumed by fire. Not surprisingly, the client felt threatened and backed off from his interactions with the dragon. When persuaded to return to this encounter, agreeing to allow his surface experience to intensify, a new experience emerged within the relationship. He began to feel very angry and unrelenting in his pursuit of the dragon, and felt as if he could destroy the dragon with fire breathed from his own nostrils. In a sense, he had become his dragon, or cancer. Thus, the dragon/cancer not only afforded him a surface experiencing, but at a deeper level it was also an appropriate target for the client's inner experience of being the cancer/dragon.

In subsequent therapeutic work, the client was permitted to begin to live out this experiencing in the session. He also began to entertain the possibility of allowing some of the associated behaviors to emerge in the extra-therapy world with other individuals who were appropriately defined as dragons. Other sessions provided him with opportunities to integrate this part of himself further. His health and oncologic status remained stable during the first month of therapy, and he returned for additional sessions.

Following similar procedures, the female client perceived a leprechaun-like trickster figure whose fundamental quality involved frustrating her by never answering a question, always joking, never being serious, and always behaving mischievously. Her experience was of extreme frustration with this figure because she wanted some straight answers from him about her health.

The experiential significance of the relationship with the trickster/cancer was that its qualities allowed her to experience frustration with being tricked by him. Nevertheless, the client's attention was fixed on this figure and she wanted to know more about him. Then, as she allowed her frustration with this character to intensify, a transformation occurred. She began to join him in playful mischievous dealings, enjoying games, tricks, and pranks. In a sense, she had become the leprechaun-like figure, a part that she had never before allowed herself to live out. She seemed to enjoy most games involving flirtation with men. In subsequent therapy she began to acknowledge these playful, mischievous qualities as parts of herself. Her breast cancer remained in remission for the first month of therapeutic work and she returned for additional sessions.

It would appear that the use of Hemi-Sync was effective with these two clients. Both felt safer and more relaxed while confronting their cancers following the tape exercise than they had in the initial stage of the session.

That vivid images representing the cancers arose while the clients perceived their cancers is not surprising. Clients who are able to encounter their diseases without first undergoing a relaxation process such as the one used here have invariably described their illness metaphorically. What is interesting is that neither approach— with or without a relaxation component—asks for figurative representations of the cancer.

It is possible that clients feel safer working with metaphorical representations than with an image of a tumor. Moreover, it is likely that the cancer is represented in this way because it and its associated image share the same experiential significance. They both display the same perceived qualities, thereby affording the same experiencing.

This approach allowed the experiential significance of the clients' cancers to be revealed, thus opening up the possibility of doing integrative work. This work illuminates the value of a powerful pathway to healing which involves becoming the "other" with which one has a dysharmonious relationship. Furthermore, evidence supporting the projection/retroflection view emerged in sessions, whereby both clients described being capable of becoming upset with people in their extra-therapy worlds who had "burned" and flirted with them, respectively. Becoming the "other" for these clients meant becoming an alienated part of their inner selves.

Working with clients who have cancer is unique because the cancer is an "other" literally existing within the self, yet which can be experienced as an external figure. In this way, projection can exhibit an internal element of self which, if we had our way, would truly exist outside the body boundary.

Given the preliminary nature of this study and the obviously small client sample, replication with a larger sample is called for. In addition, the following points should be considered in the development of a more comprehensive study.

1. A different therapist, without a knowledge of projection/retroflection as it is understood here, might not produce data supporting this position.

2. Other approaches might be as effective; hence a comparative study including multiple therapeutic avenues would be desirable.

3. Long-term follow-up of the clients is needed to determine if benefits are achieved beyond one month.

4. It is possible that the two clients were exceptional in that most others might not have allowed the introduction of Hemi-Sync to produce the effects described. There may be as yet undiscovered variables which render certain individuals more likely to benefit from the use of Hemi-Sync.

5. Other Hemi-Sync tapes may be more effective in producing the desired effect.

However, these data are suggestive. It seems to be the case that, among many other things, use of the Hemi-Sync technology is promising in that it can afford a safety zone for beginning work with elements in life that are difficult to face.

The First Step

Rita Black

Rita Black, of Richmond, Virginia, has developed a twelve-hour workshop, "The First Step," for cancer patients. In this workshop, patients' own inner resources are explored and exploited to balance and strengthen their mental attitude, release fears, and fortify their physical bodies. The workshop acts as reinforcement to medical treatment and can have the effect of limiting the unpleasant reactions to that treatment. Rita Black trained with Dr. Bernie Siegel and his Exceptional Cancer Patient Clinic and "The First Step" incorporates some of his thinking and methods.

"Motivated by strong evidence that cancer is associated with lifestyle. . ." are the opening words of the Cancer Prevention Resource Directory published by the U.S. Department of Health and Human Services. As that evidence continues to accumulate, we become increasingly aware that the human condition is the result of human thought processes, and the value of the research into human consciousness by pioneers like Robert Monroe will become more and more apparent.

My experience of Monroe's hemispheric synchronization technique was a turning point in my life, enabling me to make contact with my unseen, nonphysical self and to apply this newly uncovered personal energy. I became a Gateway Outreach trainer and began running courses in my own geographic area. Then, three years after my first visit to the Institute, my brother was diagnosed as having esophageal cancer. Only two years previously my father had died of that same disease, and the emotional wounds of that experience were not completely healed. Surely, I felt, there must be an alternative, a better way of dealing with this destructive force.

It was in a desperate effort to save my brother's life that I called upon the hemispheric synchronization process. As he listened to the taped exercises I saw how he welcomed this intensive exposure to mind expansion. We were aiming especially to shift the thought patterns connected with our father's cancer, and I tried to teach my brother everything I had learned in my own journey into self-awareness, providing him with tools to help him survive. Although the final battle was lost, there were triumphs on the way. After more than three hundred hours of highly toxic chemotherapy, my brother did not lose his hair, as the doctors predicted he would. He maintained his mental and physical stamina through eighteen sessions of radiation. Six weeks before he died, his physical strength began to wane, and he was virtually pain-free until three days before his death. It was only during his final hours, when his body chemistry was out of balance, that his mental power was unable to overcome the pain.

It was through this experience that a void in the field of cancer treatment became apparent to me. From the time the diagnosis is made until therapy begins, the patient's thoughts are chaotic. Such thoughts can actually reduce the chances of survival. Very few support systems prepare a patient for the rigorous therapy that lies ahead. Changes in lifestyle are drastic and immediate. Moreover, life-threatening illnesses affect everyone within the patient's social circle. Physical and emotional imbalances run together; anger, guilt, fear, embarrassment, and despair all add to the crisis. It is at this alarming time in the patient's life that Hemi-Sync can be of help.

I have no traditional medically-acceptable credentials and this has been a barrier for me to overcome. My natural timidity, which would have limited my vision, has had to be overcome as well. But, having determined to fill this void in treatment, I was fortunate to find several cancer patients who were willing to work with the Hemi-Sync sound technology, and from their experiences I was able to develop a twelve-hour intensive workshop. This introduces to patients with cancer and other serious illnesses the concept that they are more than their physical bodies and that, in a state of expanded awareness, they are able to recognize and use their personal internal energy systems in dealing with the disease.

Psychoneuroimmunologists tell us that stress inhibits the immune system. Our thoughts alter our brain chemistry, and negative thinking and negative reactions to external stimuli prevent our fullest participation in life. We are in danger of becoming physically entrapped by our heritage of negative and limiting thought processes. On the other hand, positive thoughts enhance the immune system, and thoughts that induce relaxation release benzodiazipine, which helps to tranquilize our bodies and minds.

"The First Step" incorporates in its program the principle that love is a healing energy which is latent within all of us, as has been demonstrated so vividly in the work of Dr. Bernie Siegel. The Hemi-Sync technology is used to help the release of habitual destructive thought processes. Participants learn to use thought-images to help in healing, through visualizations in which they explore their physical, mental, and emotional bodies. When imbalances are discovered, thought-imaging helps to correct them. Moving through the program, participants in a state of expanded awareness are encouraged to develop patterns for their lives in the future; patterning the physical body, patterning accomplishments, patterning for necessary changes one month or more ahead. This works from the basic assumption that thoughts manifest as things; that which we think, we become. Our environment is our looking-glass, reflecting back to us the shape of our thoughts.

The program evolves at each participant's own pace. Watching the energy return to an imbalanced body and seeing the "livingness" return to an otherwise hopeless human being is the reward. There is, as yet, no graph that can chart the reaction of participants and no "statistics" that can "evaluate their progress." But I recall one lady who had 80 percent of her liver surgically removed. Physically she recovered from the surgery, but emotionally she could not. Several months after she participated in "The First Step," I visited her. She was wearing a becoming wig after losing her hair from follow-up chemotherapy and she was smiling. She said "My family and I want to thank you and your program for saving my life." Hemi-Sync had given her the tools to live.

Recently I have discovered that a fellow Professional Division member of The Monroe Institute, James Greene, has simultaneously developed an almost identical program to address the HIV-positive patient. This is a dramatic verification of the merit of using this technology to regain and maintain the quality of life. Neither of us knew of the other's work until a recent professional meeting.

My personal experience confirms that crisis is a teacher. We may find ourselves in the middle of our personally created vortex and suffer because of it. Finally, when we are sick and tired of being sick and tired, and if we haven't perished in our own maelstrom, we cry out to break the barriers that confine us. Crisis can serve us well—if we are willing to listen and to learn.

Note: Typically, "The First Step" program includes listening to and discussing Monroe tapes Discovery 1, 2, & 4, Threshold 5 & 6, *and* Adventure 1, *as well as tapes from the H-PLUS series (see addendum).*

Positive Immunity

James Greene

James Greene is a businessman and educator from Arlington, Virginia. He has recently developed a program designed to help people diagnosed as HIV-positive and those who are closely involved with them. He reports as follows.

On December 17, 1987, *USA Today* published a report on a study by Mark Rider, a music therapist from Southern Methodist University, and Dr. Jeanne Achterberg, of the University of Texas Health Science Center, on the effects of creative visualization. A group of thirty volunteers listened periodically to a twenty-minute tape containing a relaxation message followed by music. They were asked while listening to visualize specific types of blood cells being released in their bodies. After six weeks, blood tests showed that the only cell count that increased was the one they had visualized.

While reading this report, it occurred to me that the combination of creative visualization and the hemispheric synchronization technology could aid in T-cell production for people who are infected with the human immunodeficiency virus (HIV). With The Monroe Institute's support, and after two years of planning, the Positive Immunity (PI) pilot program was completed in the fall of 1989. The potential health benefits are proving to be extraordinary.

During the last ten years, while medical researchers have focused on developing an HIV-positive vaccine, comparatively little was being done on the psychological level. Instead of telling people to prepare themselves to die, it seems far more appropriate to facilitate a positive attitude toward living. This way of thinking can lead to a more productive and rewarding life and may possibly help to eliminate the virus.

The PI program is not restricted to HIV-positive persons. It is intended also to help those who are living with, or who are involved with, those who have tested positive or who have full-blown AIDS.

With a goal of tapping inner guidance and healing or strengthening the immune system, the program was developed to meet the mental, emotional, physical, sleep, and total-self needs of the individual. Robert Monroe advised on the selection of a number of tapes from the Gateway Experience series. In addition, copies of the *Focus 12 Immunizing* script, specially written by Robert Rosenthal, M.D., are given to the participants. This guided imagery journey through the body's cells is specifically designed to help increase the body's T-cells, or helper cells, which are instrumental to the immune system's functioning.

Participation in the program is limited to ten people per workshop and begins with an evening orientation and two tapes. The next day includes the remaining five tapes and discussion. A full two-day program is desirable when possible. Once the group has completed the first seven exercises, I recommend using H-PLUS tapes on an as-needed basis. Several tapes of these function exercises may be useful, because people who contract the virus may develop problems to which they are genetically predisposed. They can then structure a more individualized program for themselves.

The feedback on the PI program has been generally positive. Not all participants continue to use the tapes after the workshop, but those who do report very encouraging results. To my knowledge to date, the T-cells of at least three participants have increased. Reaching HIV-positive persons before their T-cell counts plunge to a very low level and before they develop opportunistic infections seems to increase the chances of maintaining the integrity of the immune system and perhaps strengthening it.

The most difficult problem is determining exactly how beneficial the tapes are. A diagnosis of HIV-positive is almost always a life-and-death issue, making it virtually impossible to develop the participant's confidence to the extent that he or she is willing to use Hemi-Sync to the exclusion of other systems. All participants are under the care of at least one physician and are using numerous prescribed therapies. Thus, unless the facilitator is also the participant's physician, or is working directly with the physician, it is unlikely that the efficacy of Hemi-Sync can be precisely determined. My hope is that the PI program will be expanded and facilitated by physicians or certified non-medical professionals in association with physicians, which would enable us to compile more comprehensive data. Additionally, PI could become an adjunct therapy integrated with the primary health-care services being received by the participant.

I believe that the appropriate H-PLUS exercises prescribed for individuals in the early stages of immune system dysfunction can affect their longevity. Perhaps even more important, the quality of their lives can be improved through developing an understanding that they are more than their physical bodies. At this time, perhaps the only way to evaluate the PI program honestly is to put the question to the participants and trust their judgment. The testimony of one of our original participants brings this message vividly to light.

What are the things I am doing to stay well? One major thing is using the Monroe tapes. I find a combination of H-PLUS and Gateway tapes to be optimal. I believe this is because the H-PLUS tapes work for me as a direct mind-to-body experience, while the others provide me with spiritual nourishment. Jim Greene and Bob Monroe obviously recognized the benefits of both when they developed the PI program. I find two tapes especially helpful: *Restorative Sleep* (H-PLUS) and *One Month Patterning*. All, however, have something to offer, and I believe each person who uses them regularly will develop a combination that works best for him or her. Initially I used one or two tapes every day at 4 P.M.. Now I listen when I feel the need, and don't have a regular schedule. The tape I use and the time are determined by my own sense of hunger. I do, however, keep the tapes handy at all times.

Although the tapes are excellent in themselves, I believe the most important thing I have gotten from them is the ability to go into Focus 10 and Focus 12 without them, and to put my "altered state" to good use. Recently, for example, while in the dentist's chair, I was able to close out pain by using Focus 10. No tapes were involved; I merely used the technique.

What I hope I have just described is a process wherein the tapes are a support mechanism, playing a dominant training role in the beginning and a less frequent, but important, refresher role when one becomes familiar with the techniques.

Has the Positive Immunity project saved me from sickness or death? No one can know that, but I do believe it has played a significant role in my continuing state of overall well-being.

Walking the AIDS Circle

Barbara Bullard, M.A. and Kathleen Carroll, M.A.

In the fall of 1991, Barbara Bullard, a professor of Speech Communications, organized her first Positive Immunity seminar using the methods pioneered by Jim Greene. Since then, with her colleague Kat Carroll, she has developed the California Positive Immunity pilot program. What follows is a report on their findings after working with this program for two years.

When viewed as a circle, the process of birth, transformation, and death seems to present us with a series of beginnings, for nothing ever ends. However, it is not always easy to think in those terms when walking that circle as a survivor of AIDS. Birth becomes the act of simply waking up each day, transformation involves daily survival with new routines, foods, drugs, and dramatic changes in life styles, and death is a shadow constantly reminding you of how delicate life is. Working for the last two years with survivors of AIDS in the Positive Immunity Program has allowed the two of us to journey along the edge of this fragile circle called the HIV virus. It has also given us the precious opportunity to know the "peaceful warriors" who walk that circle daily.

Six years ago several of our students and friends were diagnosed HIV-positive. It was natural to apply our backgrounds in the use of sound, positive imagery, and self-healing to help our friends cope with this frightening new disease. A short time later, we discovered information about the H-PLUS tapes and added several of them to our work.

Several years later, based on the research conducted by Jim Greene and Georgetown University, we decided to embark on a "larger" AIDS circle by offering the Positive Immunity Program (PIP) in California. The PIP involves an intensive weekend incorporating tapes from Gateway I and 2 as well as an introduction to the H-PLUS tapes. It has been two years since that decision, and we are ready to share some of the lessons we have witnessed on this path of birth, transformation, and death.

First, AIDS survivors report that living with this disease is like being "reborn" into a new world—one with its own language, treatments, schedules, support systems, and opportunities. Initially, it can be a very intimidating experience and how well someone copes with the experience depends on the attitude with which he/she enters it. It is not news that attitude is a key factor in healing. We have observed this to be paramount with the AIDS survivors with whom we work. Those who resist this "rebirth" with anger or fear weaken faster and have an average survival rate of eighteen months after diagnosis. Those who embrace this "rebirth" with an attitude of hope seek alternative treatments, use the Monroe tapes more regularly, and have a longer survival rate. For example, of eight individuals participating at a recent PIP weekend, six reported that they have never used traditional drug therapies such as AZT and DDI. Using positive attitudes, nutrition, exercise, and support systems such as the Monroe tapes, this six "asymptomatic" individuals are classified as "long-term survivors," one of whom was diagnosed over eleven years ago.

Our second observation is that people who have a positive attitude about their survival enter the weekend workshop ready for healing and transformation. The PIP workshop provides opportunities for transformation to occur at all levels. During the course of two days, participants are guided through nine taped exercises. We end with a guided imagery on the immune system and encourage participants to use four additional exercises independently over the next few weeks while recording all individual insights.

Transformation begins early in the workshop. As we work with Focus 10 the morning of the program, people may experience a physical cleansing, displaying symptoms such as aching and cramping muscles, headaches, nausea, and back pain. We use massage therapists and energy workers to facilitate the cleansing of toxins from the body. We also highly encourage participants to consume water throughout the weekend to aid in this process. As we move into the Focus 12 tapes, emotional and mental shifts begin. These shifts become integrated when, at the end of the first day, we use the *Living Body Map* as a tool for unifying the physical, emotional, and mental transformations. For some individuals, the experience moves on to a spiritual transformation on the second day when we use *Free Flow 12* and an immune journey guided imagery. Anyone who has worked with the Monroe tapes knows that this level of transformation is highly individualized. However, we feel that powerful changes are occurring as evidenced by dramatic differences in complexion, muscular relaxation, and actual reduction in AIDS symptoms. One participant was suffering from KS lesions that had moved into his sinuses. He had been receiving radiation therapy, which caused the tissues around his eyes to swell severely and turn dark purple. By the end of the workshop the swelling was visibly reduced and the discoloration had shifted to pink. He exclaimed, "I can almost recognize myself when I look in the mirror!"

By the end of the second day we hear comments such as "I have never felt so relaxed," "I haven't had this much energy in months," and "I am leaving with tools that I can really use on my own—wow!" Our journey, however, does not end when these individuals walk out the door. We remain as part of their support system by continuing to monitor and mentor their use of the tapes, which includes introducing them to many of the H-PLUS tapes such as those found to be the most beneficial by former participants. (Interestingly, participants have found the *Immunizing* tape [H-PLUS] to be ineffective because the function command "attack-destroy" is not conducive to building an immune system in the face of an auto-immune disease.) In addition to "tape education" we have also offered support group meetings where we provide access to and experiences in additional alternative methods such as oxygenation therapy, rebirthing, and meditation.

Lastly, we have found ourselves walking to the end of the circle with individuals who face the final part of the cycle of life. As we sit by hospital beds or counsel grieving family and friends, the Monroe tapes are a continuous part of the process. For example, many people choose to have Metamusic playing by the bed of a dying loved one, or use it themselves as a coping tool. Following the recent death of a friend and former PIP participant, the family purchased ten tapes for their personal use. After the funeral of another participant, we watched as friends divided his "Monroe collection" up amongst other AIDS survivors. It is at moments like these when we realize the importance of "walking the circle" with someone as he moves from rebirth, through transformations, and finally finishes where he began, closing his circle and moving through death into whatever rebirth awaits him.

The experiences of the past two years have proven the value of having Hemi-Sync in walking this path. It provides coping tools for those struggling with this new way of living, it opens doors to greater human transformations, and it can be used to help create a harmonious release from a body stricken with AIDS. It certainly gives all of the "peaceful warriors" facing life with AIDS a most vital tool for their journey.

Tapes used in the Positive Immunity Program:

<u>Weekend Program</u>
Orientation Focus 3
Introduction Focus 10
Advanced Focus 10
Free Flow Focus 10
Introduction Focus 12
Energy Bar Tool
Color Breathing
Living Body Map
Free Flow Focus 12

An additional guided imagery (Immune System Journey) is used at the end of the program.

<u>Recommended tapes for continued growth</u>

Release & Recharge
Exploration Sleep
Problem Solving
One Month Patterning

<u>Recommended H-PLUS, Metamusic and Mind Food tapes</u>

<u>H-PLUS:</u>
Regenerate
Circulation
Reset
Restorative Sleep
Tune-Up
Lungs Repair & Maintenance
Off-Loading
Let Go

Metamusic:
Sleeping Through the Rain
Inner Journey
Cloudscapes
Transformations
Prisms

Mind Food:
Energy Walk

ME, PVFS, or Whatever

Jill Russell, L.C.S.P. and Ronald Russell, M.A.

Jill and Ronald Russell co-direct The Russell Centre in Cambridge, England.

What this condition is called seems to depend on whom you consult and where you are. Myalgic encephalomyelitis, Epstein-Barr syndrome, post-viral debility, post-viral fatigue syndrome, epidemic neuromyasthenia, yuppie flu, or perhaps it's "all in the mind"; but what you know is that you feel debilitated and constantly tired, suffer muscle fatigue, sometimes very painfully, after exercise of any sort, find it hard to concentrate, and are severely depressed. If you are unlucky, your doctor may not take "it" seriously, which only makes you feel worse. Whatever the diagnosis, you know—and more and more doctors are coming to accept—that something is wrong with your system and that action is needed to help to put it right.

Sufferers from this malaise—referred to as ME for the sake of brevity—may be unable to continue working and, although the condition itself is now accepted as not being a psychiatric disorder, may fall prey to mental and emotional problems. As Dr. Charles Shepherd, who has had the disease for many years, writes in his recent book *Living with ME*, "ME sufferers don't make easy patients—you've got what is probably a long-term illness that can't be "cured"; you have a wide variety of symptoms which modern medicine is very limited in its ability to help; and you may also have a whole range of social, emotional, and employment problems which require help. So, from your doctor's point of view, ME patients are not the easiest of people to manage successfully."

It is in the area of management of the condition that we wondered if Hemi-Sync might help when another therapist sent two of his female patients to see us. Susan, age twenty-six, was a finance adviser in a major bank; Yvonne, twenty-one, was an art student two-thirds of her way through a degree program. Both had been diagnosed with ME, or post-viral fatigue syndrome; both were debilitated and depressed, reporting many of the usual symptoms, lacking in confidence, and expressing little hope of recovery. Both had refused tranquilizing or anti-depressant drugs suggested by their doctors. Although they came independently, after two individual sessions we brought them together and they soon became close friends, giving each other valuable support.

We felt that the H-PLUS series might help them to handle the symptoms and to direct the body's powers of self-healing. According to Dr. Shepherd, "Rest is the most important factor in promoting recovery from ME. . .not only relaxing physically but mentally as well." We began with the H-PLUS relaxation exercise. After listening to this, one of them commented, "This is the most relaxed I've felt for years. Unlike drugs, it can only do me good." We introduced further exercises, and in addition they could make their own selection from the H-PLUS library that the Institute had provided. Later they used the first three *Discovery* exercises and joined an eight-session weekly course with exercises in Focus 10 and Focus 12.

For a time Susan used ten H-PLUS functions every day. She also developed her own function command, "Energy. . .Heal," which she used several times a day. She found *Empathizing* useful as it enabled her, it seemed, to achieve an understanding with her hospital doctor. "We were communicating beyond the spoken word," she said. She also felt that the *Discovery* tapes helped to give her security and confidence.

"The tapes provided a safe environment in which to get to know myself," she reported. "I'm feeling in control again after a period of feeling controlled by illness and doctors. These exercises give me freedom and encouragement to recognize my own needs and to use the appropriate tapes as a solution in the form of a command. . .The more you use the commands, the more they will work. . .The more I use the tapes the more I see that everyone could benefit in some way. Like me, those who do not admit it, even to themselves, are the ones who need it most. I have learned to ask for what I want and not to feel guilty about getting it. I feel stronger and happier with myself."

Yvonne found certain exercises especially useful, including *Light Foot* ("I imagine myself running—it did seem to lighten my step"), *Empathizing* ("useful for trying to understand how difficult it is for other people to cope with my illness, as well as myself"), and *Brain: Repair & Maintenance* ("very good for sharpening up my brain functions. . .it feels like I'm thinking more clearly and efficiently...It's enough to remind me how my brain used to feel and to know that sometime it will go back to being like this again"). She added:

> *Discovery 1, 2* and *3* are brilliant for confidence and to [help you] feel you can achieve things. It's as if a balance is really being found inside my mind. I guess it's putting things in proportion; important, because it's sometimes hard to live in the real world when you are isolated and living a life very different to the one you were used to...I'm very pleased with the help the tapes have given me. I'm much more in control and feel less tense and more confident...It's like re-learning the things you knew as a child—and makes me feel I'm doing things for myself—great for confidence again! It's marvelous to feel my mind isn't just a soggy lump of cotton wool, which it used to feel like.
>
> While I've been doing these tapes I've noticed that I have taken control of the situation I'm in. I used to put myself out for other people, tiring myself and then getting upset and angry. Now when I'm feeling tired, I'm learning either to go and lie down or to ask people to leave—and to my amazement they agree! Stupidly, I'd expected them to know when I was getting tired and expected them to act accordingly. My boyfriend, who has only known me since I've been ill, thinks I'm a different person now—personally I think I'm going back to what I used to be, but with a few subtle changes which have helped a lot to make me into a stronger person.

Susan and Yvonne worked with the tapes for about a year. Susan eventually left her job—she had been on sick leave for many months—and took a training in remedial massage; she now has her own private practice as well as a baby boy. Yvonne was able to return to college and complete her courses, obtaining a good degree; she is now a freelance illustrator and has had some of her cartoons published. Both have listened to all the available H-PLUS tapes and have joined the ME Society so that they can help and advise others with this condition. Susan is currently working with a small group of ME patients, using selected exercises.

Is it possible to draw any conclusions from this? With ME, as with so many other conditions, a positive attitude is very important; if you believe you can recover, the chances are far greater that you will. Susan and Yvonne learned to trust the process; they worked intensively with the tapes, never despairing when a function did not immediately click into place but persisting and seeking alternatives. While it is not possible to say how much the Monroe tapes contributed to their recovery, it is quite clear that conventional medication did nothing for them as they ceased using it. The experience does suggest, however, that occasional or casual use of the taped exercises is unlikely to be of much benefit for ME patients. Intensive use in optimum listening conditions is recommended if the process is to take effect, and this has proved to be so with other ME sufferers whom we have encountered recently.

Recovery From Closed-Head Trauma
Susan Tirotta

In 1975 Susan Tirotta was a twenty-year-old college student. She was suffering from an undiagnosed bleeding duodenal ulcer, and one day in October she fainted, hitting her head on the corner of a marble table top as she fell. No one found her, and when she came around she struggled to find help by climbing upstairs to the second floor of the college building. Halfway up she fainted again, fell to the bottom of the stairs, and lay there unconscious. Some time later she was found by a group of students, who summoned an ambulance. She was taken first to the college clinic, where she was examined and then sent on to a large medical center about twelve miles away. In the ambulance Susan had her first out-of-body experience. She found herself looking down on the ambulance attendant from above and hearing him say to the driver, "We're losing her—you'd better step on it!" Then he administered some type of injection and she returned immediately to her unconscious body. She records in her own words what followed.

In the emergency room at the medical center I experienced several disjointed out-of-body experiences. At one time I heard myself diagnosed as being in a coma. My head was shaved and two surgeons clamped my scalp together with large metal clips. When, many hours later, I regained consciousness, I was told that I had suffered a brain contusion and severe concussion. I was terrified to remain in the huge, impersonal medical center and asked to be discharged, promising to go directly to the college clinic and check myself in. But instead I returned to my dormitory and fell asleep. When I awoke I had a splitting headache and found my pillow and bedding soaked in blood. It was then I first realized that there was something very wrong with me.

A friend drove me fifty miles to my parents' home to recuperate. I was disoriented and weak as a kitten. At times I would fall suddenly into deep sleep when people were talking to me. I found it difficult to carry on a coherent conversation and would forget in mid-sentence what I had begun to say. I had forgotten how to read and write and could walk no more than fifty feet without sitting down to rest. I would suddenly begin crying for no apparent reason. Things people said to me did not make sense, and I felt out of touch with my thoughts, my emotions, and my body. I had blinding headaches, and my vision was periodically blurred. I felt as if I were having a nervous breakdown—or else going mad.

Now I tended to divide my life into "before the accident" and "after the accident." "Before" I was a gifted student, with an IQ in the range of 142 to 145. I had graduated at the top of my high school class, was popular with my contemporaries, and belonged to many clubs and athletic teams. I was a keen skier, tennis player, and equestrienne, had been accepted on scholarship to a leading university in pre-veterinary medicine, enjoyed an active and fulfilling social life, and had a loving and supportive family. Mine was a competitive, "type A" personality; in many ways I could be described as an over-achiever—and this may have been responsible for the duodenal ulcer!

After the accident, I was physically weak, out of balance, and mentally insecure. Slowly my ability to read and write returned as my brain began to heal itself. My family doctor, when he removed the metal clamps from my head, remarked that had the injury been half an inch on either side it would probably have blinded or even killed me. But the doctors who saw me knew little about "closed-head trauma" and failed to recommend either a neurologist or a physical therapist.

I felt that my mind was betraying me. Although I did not know how to remedy this, I determined to do what I could. Two years previously I had become involved with Hatha Yoga; now I turned to this in earnest, and branched out into Raja Yoga, Mantra Yoga, and Kundalini Yoga. My out-of-body experiences sparked off a deep interest in the metaphysical and spiritual areas. After several months my body and mind had strengthened enough for me to return to college, but I was a shadow of my former self.

For about three years following the accident, splitting headaches continued to trouble me. No matter how much I worked through meditation and self-discipline, I lacked confidence in my mental abilities and emotional reactions. Nevertheless, I graduated from college, began working for a living, and eventually married. But my eyesight gradually worsened; now I had to wear glasses all the time, not only for reading. Although no one else could apparently see it, I felt "damaged." Often I would have to stop in mid-sentence and try to express my thoughts in a different way. I had lost much of my earlier vocabulary. I continued to meditate daily, both alone and in groups, and to explore my spiritual path, but I had to resign myself to the fact that there were parts of my brain that would never heal.

Then, fifteen years after the accident, by what I can only describe as a "strange and serendipitous route," I came across Hemi-Sync. From a list of the tapes I ordered the H-PLUS exercise *Brain: Repair & Maintenance.* I listened to it four times before beginning to notice results. In addition to raising and showing horses, I work as an administrative assistant in a university and have to compose a lot of correspondence and reports. The more I used the "Plus Flow Better" function command, the easier it became for me to express myself both verbally and in writing. I began to look forward again to talking with other people. After three months of using the command on what I imagined to be the damaged visual center of my brain, one day I realized that I had gone throughout the day without picking up my glasses from the bedside table.

I now use this command several times daily, beginning in the shower in the morning and ending as I go to sleep at night. As I use it, it feels as if a veil is being slowly but gently lifted from my mind. I also employ the command in conjunction with various meditations on mantras, chakras, color, and light. Other exercises that I am using are *Synchronizing* and *Circulation,* as well as the *Resonant Tuning* tape. I feel that they have a cumulative effect. Although I have studied metaphysics and esoteric disciplines for many years, it is definitely the Hemi-Sync tapes which have given me back the key to my mind. I still have deficiencies in memory, emotion, and intellect that I must work continually to correct, but I feel strongly now that I can recover much, if not everything, that I "lost" fifteen years ago.

There is no medical documentation of my story. The family doctors who examined me before and after the accident are dead, and a neurological profile was never done. But I am convinced that I suffered significant brain damage which would generally be considered irreversible, especially in the light of the passage of so much time. Despite all the hardships, I am able to see the larger picture and how my life has been changed for the better by it all. I'm not sorry about my years of suffering, but I'm happy to see how I can heal myself. I hope others with similar problems will be led to use Hemi-Sync exercises when they require them and are ready to use them to the greatest advantage.

Inside, Crying Out

JoHanna Hawthorne and Susan Anton-Johnson

The experience of Susan Tirotta is paralleled in many ways by what happened to JoHanna Hawthorne, another sufferer from "closed-head trauma." The following account is adapted with permission from the book Inside, Crying Out, *by JoHanna and Susan Anton-Johnson, currently in progress.*

In January 1974, JoHanna was involved in an automobile accident. Although the car was a total wreck, she was released from the hospital after only a quick examination. There were no obvious signs of damage; no broken bones, lacerations, or loss of consciousness. There were symptoms of concussion, but these were dismissed.

Less than seven months later JoHanna was sacked from her job owing to "unacceptable performance." She had to give up a college course as she could not cope with the work. She lost her friends, and a relationship that had endured for more than a year suddenly ended. What, she wondered, had happened?

For a time she could find no answer. She cried often and uncontrollably, for no apparent reason. She found it impossible to concentrate or remember anything she read, and she could make no sense of television. When talking with others she noticed their eyes soon seemed to glaze over and it was not long before they hurried away.

JoHanna could not understand what was wrong. It was, she said, as if she were watching a movie of someone else's life. Getting lost on her way to the store, having frequent fits of anger, forgetting how to cook, shop, or wash clothes—these became commonplace. She felt as if she were living in a fog. Outside there was a world, and there was also a problem—but she had no idea that she could, or even needed to, find a solution to it.

After a year of living like this, JoHanna finally consulted a neurologist. He ran three days of painful tests and then explained the findings to her. Her brain had been organically bruised and damaged from slamming around inside her skull as a result of the severe jolting it had received in the accident. He described the injury as "closed-head trauma" and prescribed medication to stabilize the mood swings and help her to think more clearly.

At first JoHanna resisted taking the medication, but she found eventually that she could not operate without it. With its help, she began to see that the world was crumbling around her. As her confusion gradually cleared, she realized that change was essential for her life to be put back together. She understood why friends had deserted her. Although she looked as if nothing was wrong, she no longer made sense to others. In conversation, the words in her head were not the same words that came out of her mouth. She discovered also that the accident had left her operating with the social graces, and at the emotional level, of a four-year-old. This explained the mood swings—happy one minute, sad or angry the next—her short attention span, and her extreme self-centeredness. She saw a consultant psychiatrist, who diagnosed a permanent impairment of 42 percent and an intelligence impairment of 30 percent. But, like a stubborn four-year-old, JoHanna refused to accept this and vowed to get better. She refused to allow the brain injury to determine the way she lived the rest of her life.

Then began a search for tools to help JoHanna make positive changes. Once she was open to the possibility of taking action and began to discuss some of her problems, people offered suggestions of resources, books, and tapes that might help. It was as though as soon as she decided to be healthy opportunities arose to make it happen. One of these opportunities was presented by a friend who told her of the Hemi-Sync tapes. The H-PLUS series looked promising, and she ordered some of the exercises.

It was six years after the accident when JoHanna began using the tapes. Her friends soon began to notice changes. One said, "In the last two or three weeks, you've been so much brighter. You've had more energy. You've been so much quicker. Why, you're making jokes left and right!"

She was now able to work, and one day when she had made a joke a co-worker said, "Don't tell me you're brain damaged if you can make a remark that fast!" Back at her desk she recalled that she had been using the *Brain: Repair & Maintenance* exercise—and obviously it was working. Her friends and co-workers who observed how JoHanna was changing and remarked on her brightness and quickness were not aware that she was using the tapes. She herself had not realized how much she was improving until other people told her. And the only difference was that she was now listening to the *Brain* tape every night.

JoHanna found that she was sleeping better, things were going more smoothly, and breakthroughs followed one after another. There was no dramatic improvement, no overnight change, but more of an ongoing process; she handled tasks more confidently, more easily, as time went on.

Recently JoHanna has returned to her studies and gained a master's degree in Learning and Human Development Technology. She was encouraged to take NLP (neuro-linguistic programming) training and is now a certified NLP practitioner and hypnotherapist. She believes that part of knowing our capabilities is to do something that normally seems beyond our scope of possibility. With this in mind, at the end of her NLP training she was given an 11"x12"x¾" board and told to break it with her hand. Methods of concentrating and focusing to see her hand beyond the board were demonstrated, and her previous study of Tai Chi also helped. In a single swipe she broke the board without hurting her hand at all. She says that she experienced an unparalleled sense of power and assurance she had never known before, and felt that now she could do and succeed at anything she set her mind to.

"The Hemi-Sync tapes have helped in retraining my brain and recovering lost abilities to concentrate and think clearly," JoHanna says. "By practicing intensely, I've recovered my gift of music, lost at the time of the accident. Today, through words and song, I share my story at every opportunity with churches, businesses, clubs, schools, and PTAs, whenever I am asked to speak. My Higher Power has provided the opportunity to put my energy into healing and talking about my recovery. Like others in recovery, I work on healing each day, one day at a time."

Chapter 3

Well-Being

This chapter brings together reflections on various aspects of life where the Hemi-Sync technology has proved valuable. The experiences of a midwife and two mothers show how the tapes may help throughout pregnancy and during the birth process. A remedial therapist tells how she uses the technology in her practice where she treats patients of all ages and with a wide variety of conditions. There is an account of how the process helped a woman who had lost her sight. The director of a Health Rehabilitation Clinic discusses the use of Hemi-Sync in the relief of pain and stress and as an aid in relaxation therapy, and there is a detailed description of pioneering work with hospice patients. Dentists and their patients discuss their experiences with the tapes, and the chapter ends with a personal story of recovery after a near-fatal accident.

There are several other general health areas where Hemi-Sync has a contribution to make, including episodes of tachycardia, stopping smoking and other addictive habits, controlling appetite, helping the body deal with injuries and toxicity, and improving sensory perception. Work is also in progress to ascertain whether the process can help in the treatment of chemically-dependent patients, in particular those addicted to cocaine.

Pregnancy and Birth

Sheila Bick
Annemarie Young
Susanne Kuhn-Siciliano

Many women have found that the Hemi-Sync technology can prove helpful during pregnancy and the birth process. Metamusic, with its ability to create a peaceful and relaxing atmosphere, and exercises chosen from the H-PLUS series have proved especially useful. Sheila Bick, a senior midwife in a hospital in Gloucester, England, by way of experiment, offered Metamusic Midsummer Night *and* Sunset *to several selected mothers who she thought might benefit. She reported as follows.*

I would say the tapes have been very helpful in all cases, and some of my patients have been enraptured. With one patient I had to stop playing the tapes because her husband could not stay awake! In another case, I was with a woman from 1:30 P.M. until 10:00 P.M.. She found the tapes so helpful that I left them so that the next midwife could continue to play them for her. She was in the second state as I left, and I anticipated an instrumental delivery as the baby seemed big. She had a forceps delivery at 1:00 A.M.. When I went to see her the next day, the first thing she did was thank me for leaving the tapes.

Recently I looked after a lady from admission, to the Delivery Suite, to post-delivery. After I had her settled in, examined, and assessed, I made her comfortable on all fours over a bean bag. She didn't see me putting on the tape, and as the sounds drifted over she said, "Oh, what beautiful music!" I played the two tapes throughout her labor, which was fairly short. I turned the tapes off for the second stage as they didn't seem to blend with the activity of delivery. She needed an episiotomy and was really dreading the suturing. I turned on *Sunset* and we took her time getting her positioned. She just lay back, completely relaxed, while I stitched her wound. I might say I felt the benefits also.

I am completely convinced the tapes help bring about a beautiful, relaxed atmosphere which can only be beneficial. I find it interesting that many of our nurses have asked for copies, either for themselves or for relatives suffering from insomnia.

* * * * *

One mother who found Metamusic helpful during a difficult pregnancy was Annemarie Young, whose son Ben is now three years old. She began listening to Metamusic some months before he was born. The following is her story.

It helped me to relax during pregnancy, especially when I was working, which I was until six weeks before the birth was due. I was also doing Yoga for pregnancy exercises and combined these with the music.

When the time came, I took two cassettes, *Surf* and *Midsummer Night*, into the active birthroom with me. The music helped me enormously in the early stages of labor, and even later it was useful. I did, unfortunately, have a very hard time—my waters had broken before the uterus was ready and though we waited three days for labor to begin I eventually had to have an oxytocin drip. This made the contractions horrifically painful and more frequent than normal, and, as I was still not dilating, the pain was more severe. I had to have a Caesarean in the end. This was done under an epidural. So the last few hours were rather fraught, but I did find the music helped me.

My son suffered from colic for the first three months and used to cry in distress every evening for anything from two to six hours. We used to put the music on when we remembered—it wasn't always easy to remember under very fraught circumstances. It didn't work a miracle but did, I think, have a calming effect when Ben wasn't at the height of the colic pain.

Now we use the music at bedtime every night, and I'm convinced that it helps Ben sleep—or get off to sleep certainly. He likes it and listens for it when we take him up to his room—but only if he is ready to go to bed! I also find the music helps me to relax now— probably more than it did before.

* * * * *

Whereas Annemarie had no previous experience of Hemi-Sync,

Susanne Kuhn-Siciliano had taken The Gateway Experience *home course with her husband before she became pregnant with her second child. Through the program she believed that they gained a greater sensitivity to non-physical and subtle energies and were able to sense when the time was right, as she says, "to invite a little soul to be with us."*

Susanne felt that she was in touch with her son, Raphael, right from the beginning and was able to communicate with him non-verbally. However, in the second month she began to experience terrible nausea.

I couldn't keep any food in my body and I lost a lot of weight. I listened often to the *Surf* and *Cloudscapes* tapes to assist my movement into a deep state of relaxation. In that state I used my "Energy Bar Tool" [a mental tool introduced in the course] to send colored light to my troubled stomach, soothing and healing it. I experienced some very desperate days. The hours with Hemi-Sync were often the only times I felt some peace and confidence. During those deep times I felt my connection with the baby to be very strong. Non-verbally I always received the same message from him: "Don't worry about me. I'm fine. I want to be with you and I'm going to stay, no matter how stormy the sea will be." I felt a great support and strength from him during that time.

After about eight weeks the difficulties were over and I recovered very quickly. I began using tapes from the H-PLUS program. *Regenerate* and *Tune-Up* enhanced my physical well-being, and I added *Relax, Let Go, Immunizing* and *Circulation.* For the birth I introduced *Short Fix* and *Emergency: Injury.* I felt really wonderful during the last six months of pregnancy, with no heaviness or slowness. Until the last moment I was very active, running around in our vegetable garden, just loving my big belly and never feeling handicapped by it.

In the final weeks I used some of the Focus 12 patterning exercises, visualizing and feeling that we would have a wonderful in-home birth. And so it was.

When the contractions began, I started "resonant tuning" (a type of sustained vocalizing or chanting) during each wave. It was as if the tones were carrying me through the contractions, opening me up without tension or pain, and giving me energy. I was able to stay in the rhythm and the natural flow of my body. I listened to the *Surf* tape in the background and felt just great until nearly the end.

During the final stage, I had to let go of everything completely—

all tools and techniques—and simply give up. Only after that was it as if my whole being opened up and became ready to let him go. Then, there he was! So fresh, so still, slowly becoming rose-colored and opening his eyes, looking at us, very relaxed and very open.

I was up quickly afterwards and used H-PLUS *Regenerate* and *Tune-Up* regularly. My body recovered immediately. Three months after the birth I was nursing, with all the energy I needed to function normally. I attribute this to the assistance of the Hemi-Sync technology.

From my experience, and the experience of other pregnant women, I would suggest that a Hemi-Sync support program similar to mine would be of value. In the first three months of pregnancy, it is important that women be assisted in becoming accustomed to the physical changes taking place within their bodies. These changes can occur more smoothly and easily if the woman is able to relax into them, with little or no resistance. Later, after the initial physical adjustments have been made, the mother can attempt to contact her child non-verbally, using deeper states of relaxation to facilitate the contact. The patterning techniques may be used to visualize and affirm the best outcome for the pregnancy, while the H-PLUS tapes are excellent for overcoming physical problems, staying fit, and releasing emotional tensions.

It is best if, during the birth process, tapes can be played in the delivery room. If the mother chooses tapes she especially likes, those that helped her to relax during pregnancy, her body will remember the sounds and will allow her to let go more easily. If, after the birth, there is a problem due to lack of sleep, the *Catnapper* tape, which compresses a ninety-minute sleep cycle into thirty minutes, will bring refreshment to the body in a short time.

Remedial Therapy

Jill Russell, L.C.S.P.

Jill Russell is in private practice as a remedial therapist in Cambridge, England. She was a patient, and later a pupil, of Professor A.T. Andreasen, at one time Viceroy of India's Surgeon and doctor to Mahatma Gandhi. Trained in Remedial Yoga, she also employs cranio-sacral techniques where appropriate. She uses Metamusic as an accompaniment to her work and as Co-Director of the Russell Centre she helps to run courses and workshops using the Monroe technology.

I have been using Metamusic with my patients of all ages between five and eighty-five for over six years. They come with a variety of conditions, among them muscular strains, "bad backs," aftereffects of stroke, Parkinson's disease, arthritis, and rheumatism. With an auto-reverse player, the music runs continuously throughout the session. There is no doubt that it helps patients to relax much more quickly and to become receptive to treatment without delay. Indeed, the house is virtually bathed in Metamusic and most visitors seem to move into a "Focus 10 state" within a minute or two of entering the door.

From the beginning I noted a marked reduction in the more obvious kinds of stress and the quick cessation (with only one or two exceptions) of trivial chatter. The tranquil, relaxed state enables patients to move away from the fuss and bother of everyday life and into contact with deeper levels of self. The music affects me similarly, so that I am able to meet the patient on the same level where we can work together throughout the session. Communication between us opens up; the problems that underlie the physical symptoms come to the surface and are given voice. As the patient's level of consciousness shifts, as it might from Focus 10 to Focus 12, I am able to follow and to accompany her on her journey into her own inner world. My hands stay on the patient but I do nothing; I share the experience and that is all.

I find the Monroe tapes to be a resource of the highest value. Many patients have sleeping difficulties, and almost all of them have responded well to *Sound Sleeper* or *Super Sleep*. Those with long flights or rail journeys ahead of them will borrow *Catnapper* to help them enjoy periods of refreshing sleep. Where there are specific problems or difficulties, we look for an appropriate H-PLUS Function exercise for them to use at home. This enables them to take responsibility for tackling their own problems.

Sometimes it is not their problems but someone else's that patients are concerned about. One lady, an art therapist, borrowed Metamusic tapes to use with autistic and severely handicapped children and was delighted with the response. A child with whom she had worked for months made eye-contact for the very first time; another, who customarily painted in dark colors, began to use light greens, blues, and reds. Some patients borrow tapes for family members or friends, usually Metamusic or specific H-PLUS exercises. The *Concentration* tape is also in demand, as might be expected in Cambridge, a city with so many of its citizens involved in education.

For those who wish to look further into the process I suggest the first three tapes in the *Discovery* series, and many who try these go on to take workshops or courses with exercises in Focus 10 and Focus 12, while some continue with the process by traveling to Virginia for The Gateway Voyage course.

My own intuition and observation, coupled with the feedback that patients provide, guide me in the choice of the appropriate tape and enable me to assess its effectiveness. Feedback is especially helpful. "The first, almost immediate effect is relaxation of body," commented one lady on the Metamusic tapes. "Then a quieting of the mind that leads to inner stillness. So the overall effect becomes a general serenity. These tapes are a great aid to massage from the patient's point of view, giving a greater sense of relaxation and well-being."

Another patient, who borrowed tapes to use at home to supplement treatment, reported, "I have found the sleep exercise invaluable; it almost always sends me to sleep about halfway through, and though I awaken when it ends and I remove the headphones, I always get back to sleep almost immediately. I find Bob's voice comforting, a familiar voice like a friend, and I have a very real sense that he is there. I have also been very depressed and have found *Discovery 2* extremely helpful for relaxing and obtaining peace of mind."

One of my youngest patients is Victoria, age five, who was born slightly brain-damaged resulting in bone deformities in hips and legs and a number of minor mental handicaps. When she first came, her legs were in plaster casts and she was unable to walk upstairs. (She is now, thanks to cranio-sacral treatment, very much improved, and has recently been accepted by a new school as a "normal child.") Metamusic played softly during treatment seemed to release in her—and in me—a capacity for story-telling, and I began to realize that in our shared stories she was expressing emotions resulting from distressing experiences in her earlier years. Her house, she said, was "full of dust"; I knew perfectly well that the house she lived in was spotlessly clean, and it was from another "house" that the dust had to be swept away. When we told stories of giants, she spontaneously called hers "Giant Cutaleg"—a significant reference to early unpleasant experiences in the hospital. Now, thankfully, the house is clean and the giant no longer threatens.

Victoria's mother has been using Metamusic with her daughter and son John, age four, for eighteen months. Sleep, relaxation, and concentration are all improved, and John discovered he was able to read aloud fluently for the first time while a music tape carrying a relaxation-inducing signal was being played.

To sum up, I believe that the Hemi-Sync process is of much value in helping people, whether they are patients or not, to integrate body, mind, and spirit and to maintain a balance between the three. For my part, it has enabled me to work at a more profound level and to share experiences with my patients in a way that I had never thought was possible.

"Will I See Like Normal People See?"

Patricia Leva, R.N., M.A.

Patricia Leva is the founder of Natural Learning Systems in Solon, Ohio. She is also a registered nurse and an Outreach trainer for The Monroe Institute.

Sally Kubrik, now thirty-seven, was blind from the day she was born. A premature baby, she was placed in an incubator, but a fault occurred in the administration of oxygen, causing retrolental fibroplasia (burned tissue formed and covered the retina), resulting in blindness. Until recently she was unemployed and lacked direction and interest in life generally.

In August 1989, Sally heard a broadcast interview describing the use of hemispheric synchronization. She telephoned me, suggesting that this might help her improve her self-confidence and expand her attention span. On my first house call, however, I found myself floundering in my explanation, searching for words, aware that these products were by no means easy for blind folks to use. I could not draw diagrams to explain the process and I was concerned that Sally would not be able to remember one tape from another, with more than two hundred choices available, and I could not rely on the catalog to reinforce my explanation. Nor was any braille system available.

On my second visit I decided to drop the traditional, intellectual diagnostic approach. I turned to Sally and said, "You take me into your world and guide me." I listened carefully to her health-care history, highlighted by diabetes and narcolepsy first diagnosed in high school. It seemed to me that the best thing I could do was to help her with her scattered energy and poor self-esteem, so I introduced her to the H-PLUS exercises *Attention* and *Off-Loading*. She also began using *Concentration* in the evenings when sleepiness often overwhelmed her and her medication failed to take effect. By now she was working daily in a broadcasting studio as a student, and to help with this she took on exercises to improve her confidence in speaking and to help her control her mood.

Sally's mother, however, was skeptical and had reservations about the results. In Sally's own words: "I began to feel very anxious. I used the encoding 'plus fade, fade,' on the *Off-Loading* exercise and found myself minutes later saying very emphatically through my tears that I wanted to get back the eagerness for life I had as a little child. Maybe it was how I said this, but from then on it was my mother who kept noticing little things about me that were changing. And changes there were. When I used *Attention* it was as if someone opened up the top of my head, breathed fresh air inside and all of my senses snapped open!"

One significant event happened when Sally's pastor asked her to give the Palm Sunday's children's homily on "blessed are the blind" and describe to them what it was like to be blind. He also asked her to sing a favorite song of hers to the congregation. During her talk, she used the H-PLUS functions she had learned. "Having taken singing lessons for a long time," she said afterwards, "it was amazing to feel my breath control ability expand like an endless balloon. I had to use hardly any stagger breaths to regain control. I just kept talking smoothly and evenly and with ease, whereas in the past I would not have had the courage or the words to do this."

Several months later, Sally was diagnosed with carpal tunnel syndrome and surgery was advised. Having had two previous operations in the past year which caused weight loss and hypoglycemic episodes and added to her feelings of losing inner control, Sally began to dread the surgery. She asked if she could use the Emergency Series and gained the support of her orthopedist, anesthesiologist, and nursing team. She followed the recommended approach, using each exercise at the appropriate time. She managed to negotiate a local surgical intervention, rather than general anesthesia, and afterwards experienced significantly less pain, used no pain medication for the first six hours, and ate heartily in the recovery room without nausea, vomiting, or cyclic constipation. She experienced no loss of weight, as she had after earlier operations, and at the first dressing change her surgeon remarked how clean and clear her suture line looked, it being unusual for diabetics to heal so fast and well. Overall, Sally expressed a great deal of pride in being more of a partner in her own healing process.

Following this episode, Sally asked to begin on the home study series of exercises for her own inner growth. She worked with and without the tapes to become accustomed to the Focus 10 state, and found herself experiencing moments of precognition and intuitional experiences that convinced her that she was "seeing" more than she had ever looked for. This kind of intuitional skill, she thinks, might be a distinct advantage for other blind people to develop.

After a year of our working together, Sally found that she had overcome her fear of the outer world. She now looks for places to go to and recently discovered that she could understand and enjoy "watching" a game of soccer despite her blindness. "My concentration and ability to enjoy what is happening about me have increased considerably," she said. "I sleep through the nights now, usually waking refreshed, unlike a year ago when my inner anxiety continued while I was sleeping and woke me several times during the night. I feel I've grown in overall confidence and self-esteem in this past year. I'm well on the way to completing my radio broadcasting course and am looking forward to employment next summer."

Pain, Stress & Hemi-Sync
Ralph J. Luciani, D.O., M.S., Ph.D.

Dr. Ralph Luciani is the founder and director of the Albuquerque Clinic for Pain, Stress, and Health Rehabilitation in New Mexico, established in 1988. The clinic uses a multi-disciplinary approach to the treatment of chronic diseases and pain syndromes, and practices clinical preventative medicine. There is a strong emphasis on assisting individuals to make transformational shifts from thinking about physical infirmity solely as a physical phenomenon to self-realization of the inner potential of mind and spirit.

Since 1988, when Dr. Luciani and his wife Karen attended courses at The Monroe Institute, the Hemi-Sync process has played a major role in the practice of the clinic because, as Dr. Luciani says, "of its tremendous potential for effecting transformational change. It seemed to me that the process was able to aid people to get 'unstuck' and out of thinking of themselves as victims of their physical realities."

A principal use of Hemi-Sync is in the clinic's two-week intensive pain program, in which the patient spends most of each day at the clinic seeing various practitioners for therapy. Between two and three hours a day are spent in Hemi-Sync biofeedback therapy. A handbook, including a schedule of Hemi-Sync tapes, guides patients through the program, which is designed to lead them through an evolution of consciousness during the physical aspects of their therapy. During each tape-listening session, a thermistor is attached to the patient's finger to track temperature changes as an indication of the relaxation response. Each patient also receives homework tapes daily and a sleep tape each night.

The results have been quite astounding. In all cases, skin temperature rises, sometimes quite dramatically, indicating a deep level of relaxation. An interesting example was a patient who to begin with was very resistant to the idea of the tapes but continued to listen to them as directed. She admitted that, although she thought it sounded like "crazy stuff," the tapes helped her to get pain relief and to relax. At the end of her program she bought several tapes for herself and she has since reported that at the end of a stressful day she chooses one to listen to and has been able to prevent her back from hurting.

Another patient, a Vietnam veteran, was suffering from a work-related injury of two years' duration. He also had a history of Post-Traumatic Stress Disorder. During Hemi-Sync therapy he obtained insights into some of the factors that prevented him from letting go of his pain. Several scenarios from his Vietnam days were revealed to him which helped him understand himself better and feel more relaxed. Within three days of the beginning of his two-week program, all of the therapists remarked how he had already changed. He was physically less tense and his face was softer, more cheerful, and less stressed. Later he attended an Excursion workshop to explore further his emotional and physical pain.

Another area in which Hemi-Sync has proved successful is in aiding patients to stop smoking. The clinic's smoking program consists of behavioral counseling, a choice of acupuncture or hypnotherapy treatment, and the daily use of the *De-Hab Smoking* tape. All of the patients have managed to quit smoking and all report that the tape is a key factor.

A local dentist sometimes refers patients to the clinic for assistance with dental analgesia. The patient is given the *Pre-Op* tape from the Emergency Series to listen to daily for one week prior to the dental procedure. During dentistry, the *Intra-Op* tape is played, and acupuncture is administered for analgesia.

Of three patients who have recently been referred, the first was a nurse who had tremendous fear of dental pain and refused pain-killing injections. She was to have an inlay and a crown procedure—both generally considered especially uncomfortable. She experienced no pain and reported feeling totally relaxed and happy in the dentist's chair.

The second patient had a previous negative experience in dentistry with an acute hypertensive episode accompanied by agitation which required paramedical assistance. It was unclear whether the episode stemmed from extreme fear or was a reaction to the local anesthetic. Whichever it was, it was evident that an alternative was needed. She was to have extensive work: a three-unit bridge and inlay and a four-unit bridge were all to be accomplished during two separate visits. In both visits, the same treatment with Hemi-Sync and acupuncture was used. The patient said that one area in her right anterior mandible remained a bit sensitive, but she endured both visits with minimal discomfort and no agitation. She did not want her earphones removed even after the acupuncture was discontinued, and noted that the tape helped her to feel at ease and detached from discomfort.

The third patient was an extremely environmentally sensitive woman who could not tolerate drugs or anesthesia of any kind. She needed several fillings and, following the same program as the others, completed the treatment with minimal to no discomfort.

Two patients in recent months who needed surgery used the Emergency Series. The *Pre-Op* tape was given to them a few days beforehand for daily listening. One patient, due for a hysterectomy, was able to listen to *Intra-Op* during her operation. In the recovery room and for several days thereafter she used the *Recovery* and *Recuperation* tapes daily. She required minimal self-administered analgesia on the first day and virtually no medication afterwards. The nursing staff encouraged her not to be stoical and to use medication when she had pain. However she insisted she had little or no discomfort and was discharged on the third day.

The second patient, diagnosed with a ruptured disc, underwent a lumbar laminectomy. She reported very little need for pain medication after the surgery and was released from the hospital much sooner than expected. She was delighted, as was the hospital staff, at her fast recovery rate.

Metamusic and other tapes used with Hemi-Sync signals are also played at the clinic during massage therapy, acupuncture treatment, and relaxation training. During massage therapy, the music over open speakers not only allows the patient to relax but also supports the therapist in achieving a deeper insight into the patients' problems. During acupuncture, patients reach a deeper state of consciousness which enhances the energetic acupuncture therapy.

In conclusion, the use of the Hemi-Sync process has proved to have significant clinical use for various problems from pain management to relaxation therapy. Its uses are limited only by lack of application. Wherever and whenever the integration of body, mind, and spirit is a therapeutic goal, Hemi-Sync can be of invaluable assistance.

Hemi-Sync In the Hospice

Ruth Domin

Until her death in 1989, Ruth Domin was Director of Volunteers and Education at a hospice in southeastern United States. The hospice is a non-profit agency providing specialized home care for patients in the last stages of life-threatening illness. Nurses, other health professionals, and a corps of trained volunteer patient- and family-support practitioners address problems of pain, fear, anxiety, and loneliness in order for the end of life to be experienced as a natural event within the warm environment of the family. In 1986 the hospice began to investigate the potential of the Monroe technology with selected patients, and Ruth Domin reported on progress with sixteen of these patients in the following year.

The purposes of using the Hemi-Sync tapes were to alleviate pain and the memory of it; to relieve personal or intrapersonal stress associated with life-threatening disease, death or dying; to free the spiritual elements of the physical forces of the body; and to bring ease, comfort, and harmony to patients and their families. Careful procedures were established to ensure that nurses and support practitioners who monitored the tapes were familiar with them and used them for their own benefit, and that tapes were offered to patients as an option to help control their symptoms. Small stereo cassette players and headsets were provided for patients who did not possess them.

Before a tape was introduced, the patient's nurse described the process and its possible benefits. The Director of Volunteers and the support practitioner accompanied the nurse on the first occasion the tape was to be used. The patient's vital signs were monitored before, during, and after the first use of the tape, and a notebook was left with the patient or the primary family caregiver for keeping a record of the date, time, and response for each session. The nurse checked the notebook each week and discussed the patient's reactions to the tape, while the support practitioner also visited weekly to discuss the tape with the patient and the caregiver and to monitor the patient during tape use. Both the nurse and the support practitioner filed reports which were discussed at team meetings to establish plans for patient care. Where appropriate, tapes were also offered to the primary caregivers to use for their own benefit.

It was found that the patients who benefited most were those who trusted easily, responded well to suggestion, were not receiving total effectiveness from medication, disliked sedation and the side-effects of medication, and desired an alternative to the use of drugs. Those who were able to integrate new ideas into their own beliefs and practices also benefited. Neither age nor religious affiliation, nor the lack of it, were important factors in the successful use of the tapes. Among the patients who were helped were a "backslidden" Baptist, an agnostic, a Church of God minister, a sixty-five-year-old Seventh Day Adventist, and a thirty-five-year-old mother with no religious affiliation.

Nurses found that it was important to ensure a trusting relationship with the patient and family before introducing a tape; it also helped to be aware how the patient coped with stress and to evaluate what was going on with the patient during the day. Setting goals for the tapes helped, especially asking the patient "What are your needs?" and determining the symptoms to be managed. It was necessary to listen to the patient carefully to establish the goals; in one case what the patient really wanted was more energy, but the assumption had been pain control. It was also important to ensure a quiet, orderly environment for listening, with no interruptions if possible.

Nurses learned to introduce tapes gently and cautiously, checking on patients' preferences and practices. When one lady was asked if she had heard of guided imagery, she said "Is that like seeing things? Sometimes the devil sits on my shoulder. I go to the door and open it. Then I tell the devil to go. I close the door and he's gone." She was told that was a good example of guided imagery and she used the tapes quite successfully for the relief of symptoms.

Nurses discovered also how important it was to know the tapes well themselves so that they could understand what patients were talking about when they expressed their reactions. If new symptoms developed they had to be alert to summoning the appropriate support. If a tape was rejected, they needed to know why and to allow the patient to decide whether another tape might help.

Follow-up visits were vital in determining whether tape use was achieving the goals set by the patient. They were also valuable for encouraging the patient and counseling the family when a patient complained of symptoms but had little inclination to do anything about them. At times action might be needed, such as a call to a physician for permission to use a tape during the administration of chemotherapy.

Several family caregivers used the tapes to help reduce their own frustration and anxiety, while some support practitioners used them to help them sleep and to reduce blood pressure. One used the Emergency Series when undergoing eye surgery, which resulted in pain reduction and shortened recovery time.

The hospice found that use of the tapes was determined as much by the availability of people trained to administer them and work with patients as by the number of patients who could benefit. There was also a limitation imposed by time, as nurses generally were too busy to monitor the use of tapes every week.

Their experience with the Monroe technology led the hospice to submit certain recommendations to any other hospice which might consider using this process.

1. A person on the hospice team who uses the tapes and is familiar with them should be nominated to assume responsibility for tapes and equipment loaned to patients, to co-ordinate staff and volunteers to work with patients and families, and to maintain contact with The Monroe Institute.

2. Knowledge of individual patient/family belief systems is a prerequisite. Since the Hemi-Sync process lends itself to all people without regard to customs and mores, the tapes can be explained in terms each patient understands. The important factor in introducing a tape is to see the world as the patient sees it.

3. Use positive reinforcement, avoiding negative statements and words. For example, to say "The tapes have been used for pain" is to keep "pain" in mind. To say "The tapes have been used to relieve symptoms and make patients more comfortable" is to reinforce thoughts of relief and comfort.

4. Know how well a family is coping with death before offering a tape that encourages a patient to "let go." (A nurse and a social worker at the hospice noted how an elderly mother near death was "hanging on." They explained to her daughters that their mother was hanging on because she thought her children needed her. One daughter talked to her mother and gave

her permission to "let go." The mother died soon afterwards. However, a son who heard what his sister said became extremely angry. "That was a terrible thing to say to mother!" he raged. "She would be afraid." Conclusions about where the fear really lay would have done little good if the son had taken the nurse and social worker to court for urging his sisters to help his mother to die.)

5. Expect varied responses from different patients and from the same patient at different times. A tape may trigger an unexpected response in a patient.

Three Case Studies

J.M. had hemorrhaged and had been hanging on near death for many weeks. He listened to *Deep Ten Relaxation* once only. The next day, his nurse reported that he was beginning to die, which he did two days later. When the tape had been first mentioned to the sister with whom he lived, she was reluctant to permit it to be used. However, at the funeral she sought out the nurse and thanked her.

The hospice program provides a one-year bereavement follow-up period, during which the family is contacted regularly as needed. At the end of a year, a social worker visits for a closing assessment. When the social worker contacted J.M's sister at the end of the year, the sister talked again about the tape, saying that she thought it was the best thing that had happened to him. "He couldn't let go, and the tape helped him let go and die in peace."

G.W. was a patient who gave the nurse and support practitioner some challenging moments. He and his wife were both receptive to the *Deep Ten Relaxation* tape. The goals were effective pain control without increasing medication and relief of depression. The patient responded well, falling asleep the first time he listened to it. In the following days he often asked his wife to bring it to him, "even when he wasn't hurting."

However, as his physical condition deteriorated, he suddenly refused the tape and all medication. One day the support practitioner found him naked, rolling around on the bed in a darkened room, moaning "My soul is burning, burning, burning. . ." His distraught wife said he alternately asked for all of his pain medication at once or refused to take any of it.

According to his wife and daughter, the trouble began when he first heard what he thought to be a train on the tape. "At first the tape helped a lot," his wife said. "Then he got to another stage. . .he hates to let go. . .he told me, 'I don't like that damn music.' His mother said he ran away when he was sixteen. He hopped a freight train. He used to hobo around. He told me a little about it when we were first married. I think something bad happened but I don't know what."

The support practitioner asked G.W.'s wife if she thought her husband might like to talk to another support practitioner who was an evangelist. The wife was reluctant, so the support practitioner brought in the nurse who administered pain medication, prayed with G.W., talked with his wife, and, finally, in some desperation, called in the Director of Volunteers.

The Director brought the evangelist with her. At first the evangelist sat quietly by the bed. Then she asked G.W. what was bothering him. To begin with, he was noncommittal. Then ensued forty-five minutes of heated talk, Bible reading, and prayer. When the evangelist left, G.W. was resting quietly and his wife was crying tears of gratitude.

Next day G.W. asked to see the evangelist again but before his wife could contact her the preacher from the wife's church walked in. Hitherto G.W. had refused to talk to the preacher, but this time he consented and, according to his wife, "he accepted Jesus." From then on until he died a few days later, G.W. was at peace. His funeral was conducted by the preacher both of them had come to trust.

The Hemi-Sync tape had in some way brought about a crisis which led to resolving G.W.'s problem. The nurse commented to the support practitioner, "We had been working on the tip of the iceberg with medication—you uncovered the iceberg."

(A word of caution: If considering a procedure similar to that followed for G.W., please note Recommendations 2 and 5 above. An important factor in supporting a patient using a tape is to see the world as the patient does.)

V.F. was still living when this report was compiled. A seventy-two-year-old widow living alone, she had lost two husbands to cancer and has had it herself for eleven years. She first developed breast cancer, then cancer of the colon, and then metastasis to the liver, which was her condition when she was admitted to the hospice in May 1986. "I know I may die at any time," she told the social worker. "I won't give up. I like living, and I'm not going to rush it."

A nurse referred V.F. to the Director of Volunteers for possible use of a relaxation tape when she complained of nervousness but preferred not to take large doses of tranquilizers. "I have never been a nervous person," she said, "but I've been walking the floor since the chemotherapy." She was introduced to *Deep Ten Relaxation* and the following week she reported, "I haven't been taking as many pills since I began listening to the tape. I was taking one pill every four hours or less. Yesterday I took only one pill all day. I know the tape is helping me."

It was suggested that V.F. used the tape at night in bed, and she agreed to try this. She also tried visualization both with and without the tape. "Sometimes I just close my eyes and hear the voice telling me to relax—and I feel better." She had never heard the sound of surf in her life and had never seen an ocean. But when the *Surf* tape was suggested as an alternative to *Deep Ten* (which had "too much voice" for her at the time) she was willing to try it. Although nervousness and restlessness were two of her frequent complaints, she lay quietly after first hearing this tape, finally opening her eyes and saying "I'm too relaxed to move."

Eventually the surf sound needed a supplement—some commentary to help her feelings of weakness. She tried *Energy Walk* and was delighted with it. She took her cassette player with her to chemotherapy and at night when she could not sleep she walked around with her player, listening through headphones.

V.F. recorded her use of the tapes in her notebook. Here are two of her more recent entries:

"I played the tape twice today and it quieted my nerves. Not only does it help and relax me, I feel that something is happening in my body and I know it is doing something for me."

"I played the tape again today and counted my breathing with my hand over the cancer. It does something and makes me feel all over better and relaxed. I went off to sleep."

The hospice has learned much from V.F.—and indeed from every patient who has used the tapes. Both staff and volunteers feel that Hemi-Sync and hospice are a natural partnership. We hope that the method outlined above may provide a useful protocol for other hospices that may be interested in this non-invasive approach.

As a consequence of Ruth Domin's pioneering work, The Monroe Institute, with the advice of experts including Charles Tart, Ph.D., and Dr. Elisabeth Kubler-Ross, has recently completed a set of six taped exercises, specifically for use in hospices and by those involved in any way with the dying process.

Dentistry

Robert C. Davis, D.D.S.
Christopher W. Beckner, D.D.S.
Dental Patients

The use of Hemi-Sync in dental practice is on the increase. It may be made available to patients to help them relax in the waiting room or they may listen to tapes while treatment is taking place. This section includes accounts from two dentists who have recorded their patients' experiences while listening to tapes and from three patients who used them while undergoing extensive treatment.

Dr. Robert C. Davis, of Erlanger, Kentucky, documented twenty cases of patients drawn at random from his list, the only requirement being expression of interest and willingness to participate. With most of them he used conscious sedation or local anesthetic and either the Pre-Op *tape from the Emergency Series or a Metamusic tape. Notes of seven of these cases follow.*

1. A middle-aged man, recently unemployed, had postponed dental treatment for over twenty years, earlier treatment having, he said, proved unsatisfactory emotionally and psychologically. Now he felt that his employment prospects would be improved if he was more aesthetically presentable, and he was interested in an alternative approach.

On his first two visits he used the *Pre-Op* tape and also asked for a local anesthetic. His first response was "I only felt a little pain, not bad, mind you. I'll be back." After the second visit he claimed he didn't feel a thing, nor did he on the third visit, when he did not ask for anesthetic and had four teeth prepared for crowns. His final comment was "If I knew about this, I would have been here much sooner. I'll never wait this long again."

2. A man in his mid-thirties admitted a morbid fear of the needles used in dental treatment and who had postponed for too long. During

his two visits he listened to the *Pre-Op* tape. Several large restorations were completed and a tooth was prepared for a crown. He reported no pain and concluded by saying that there was nothing to be afraid of.

3. A middle-aged professional woman needed treatment quickly, requiring a longer-than-usual appointment. She used the *Pre-Op* tape and local anesthetic while several teeth were prepared for crowns. Her comment was "I can't believe I've been here so long. The time just flew by."

4. A street-wise teen-aged male had a dramatic aversion to dental treatment in general and to injections in particular. He was present as an alternative to the prospect of severe bodily harm promised by his parents (the dental insurance was due to expire shortly). He listened to Metamusic while two large restorations took place. He commented, "That's weird, I mean man, that's weird. Really weird." On the treatment he made no comment at all.

5. A boy, whose mother used the Hemi-Sync tapes, had no history of dental fears or phobias. He also listened to Metamusic while two moderately large restorations were placed, commenting that everything was fine. "I could have stayed for an hour if you wanted me to."

6. A physician in his late fifties had undergone previous dental treatment without any local anesthetic. He was interested as his family used Hemi-Sync and he listened to Metamusic while a tooth was prepared for a crown. "General anesthesia would be more effective," he said, "but outside of that. . ."

7. A patient who provided the most complex and challenging case in this study had a history which went back several years. He was a well-educated man in his mid-thirties, suffering severe stress from work-related activities. For many years he had been given Elixir Donnatal half an hour before treatment as well as extensive local anesthetic, but he never found this satisfactory although the "pain" could be tolerated. I gave him the *Pre-Op* tape to use at home in the days before treatment and he used it again, together with local anesthetic, during the visit when multiple crowns were prepared. After treatment he commented, "I'm not afraid any more, and I can sleep the night before I come to see you. I've quit taking Valium before going to work; I just play the tape."

For the most part, dentists venture forth to work in an unmarked emotional and psychological minefield, without knowing how to defuse them. This is at least a beginning. Hemi-Sync seems to be the decisive factor in enhancing the effect of both local anesthetic and conscious sedation. The patients' comments were all highly positive and there were no cases where the patient was not impressed in some manner. Could it be that Hemi-Sync alone can be adapted to meet the needs of patients, regardless of their degree of fear, phobia or anxiety, without any chemical intervention?

The first effort has accomplished more than was dreamed possible. Subsequently, this has become a standard operating procedure in my practice of dentistry.

* * * * *

Dr. Christopher W. Beckner is a dentist in practice in Hamilton, Ohio. He specializes in periodontics, the treatment of gum diseases, and he is also a certified hypnotherapist, using hypnosis with dental treatment to promote patient relaxation. Here he reports on a study of twenty-five patients using a Metamusic tape to reduce anxiety.

As a dentist, I am interested in providing the best possible health care for patients. As a hypnotherapist, I would like to teach people how to relax. Unfortunately, for many individuals relaxation and the dental visit are mutually exclusive concepts. Because of this, I continually look for ways to make the dental appointment less traumatic. If I can achieve this, my patients will be happier and my day will unfold much more smoothly.

One of the greatest stressors for the dentist is the fearful patient. Researchers estimate that more than half the population is not receiving regular dental care. Fear of the dental visit is a significant factor. Even many of those who visit the dentist regularly have at least some degree of apprehension. Hence I am interested in evaluating any non-invasive tools which may help reduce patient anxiety.

Recently I embarked on a study to observe and evaluate the effects of a Hemi-Sync tape on patient anxiety during dental treatment. I selected *Sleeping Through the Rain* for several reasons. First, it contains only music, and I felt it would be simple to coordinate it with a thirty-minute appointment. Second, the low bass tones in this piece are excellent for drowning out the sound of the dental equipment, such as the handpiece, ultrasonic scaler, and suction machine. Third, it is my favorite and I could recommend it highly. The musical composition is particularly relaxing and the frequencies integrated within the music are designed to lead the listener into a deeply relaxed state.

During a five-month period, thirty patients were given the oppor-tunity to use the tape during their appointments. I selected as potential subjects patients I perceived to be comfortable with or receptive to the use of headphones. Teenagers and young adults were eager to participate while many older adults declined. I explained that I was conducting research on the effects of music on the experience of a dental visit. I gave details of the technology only to those patients who specifically requested them. Of the thirty patients asked, twenty-five agreed to participate. Interestingly, three of those who declined tended to be extremely anxious and tense during their appointments. They wanted to remain fully alert and "in control" during the procedure and apparently feared that becoming too relaxed might prevent this. The other two, however, were able to relax on their own.

The treatment performed with the twenty-five subjects was either periodontal scaling and root planing or periodontal surgery. Both procedures are done with a local anesthetic. Appointments lasted from one-half to two hours. It was rarely necessary to employ any pharmacologic form of sedation, although occasionally nitrous oxide (laughing gas) was used.

After their appointments the subjects were asked to give their subjective opinions and impressions of the tape. I recorded my observations of each patient's behavior during treatment. While responses naturally varied, the results can be loosely divided into three categories: (1) patients who experienced their attention being distracted from the procedure; (2) patients who experienced deep relaxation; and (3) patients who experienced neither distraction nor relaxation.

Category (1) was the largest group, with twelve patients. They reported enjoying the tape because it allowed them to focus their attention elsewhere while their mouths were being worked on. Comments included that the tape "helped to take my mind off the treatment," and that it helped to cover the sound of the dental instruments. My observations of this group in general were that they appeared fairly relaxed and would alternate between having their eyes open and shut during the appointment.

Category (2), with eight patients, primarily experienced deep relaxation. They reported enjoying the tape tremendously, describ-ing it as "very relaxing" and "a pleasure to listen to." They loved the music and were outspoken in their praise of it. Two of them fell asleep during the procedure, while others commented that the tape evoked emotions. I observed that in general this group remained physically relaxed throughout the treatment and mostly kept their eyes shut.

Category (3), five patients, experienced no apparent effect. Comments included that the tape was "too boring" or "all right." Two, in their early teens, did not listen to the tape at all. Two kept their eyes open throughout the procedure and their bodies remained tense. They said that the tape made no difference one way or the other.

There are two main ways in which patients can effectively cope with the experience of dental treatment: relaxation and distraction. People who have learned to relax and distract themselves have a distinct advantage in dealing with some of the less pleasant aspects of life. In my experience as a dentist, I have noticed that only about 20 percent of my patients have cultivated effective relaxation or distraction techniques which appear to promote relaxation and comfort during dental procedures. The remainder continue to demonstrate or express some degree of tension or anxiety. In this informal study the reverse occurred: 80 percent reported feeling relaxed or distracted with the tape, and only 20 percent reported no effect. My observations of their behavior corroborate their subjective statements. So, although I am not attempting to draw any conclusions from the results of the study, it is clear that the use of the tape had some positive impact on the experience of dental treatment.

Recently I had some dental work done myself and, having not had dental treatment for some time, I must admit it was very enlightening. Suddenly I was the patient. The procedure itself was painless. I knew exactly what was being done and was not particularly nervous. Also I am fairly adept at relaxation and self-hypnosis techniques. Nevertheless, I found it difficult to relax and, without a tape to listen to, I was on my own. As I attempted to concentrate on relaxing my body, my attention was drawn to the sound of the drill and the work being done on my tooth. Thinking to myself "This is a challenge to relax in the dental chair," I would have given anything to be "sleeping through the rain."

I will continue to offer the tape to patients and fully intend to take my headphones with me to my own next appointment.

* * * * *

Patients' Experiences

Many dental patients have testified as to the effectiveness of various Hemi-Sync tapes during treatment. One of these, Eileen, about to have a crown prepared, a filling, and cleaning in the same appointment, refused anesthetic despite the dentist's warning that there would be a lot of exposed nerves, gum manipulation, and major drilling involved. She preferred to use self-hypnosis and the *Pain Control* tape. She felt the sensations throughout the procedure but registered no pain at all until several hours later when, feeling pain on the opposite side of the mouth from where the work had been undertaken, she discovered that she had cut herself on the bitewing used for an x-ray.

Eileen had two more crowns fitted a few months later. On the first occasion, she again used the tape but was distracted by the dentist talking with his assistant and was aware of the sensation of pain although it was not severe. Next time she asked the dentist to talk as little as possible, and she used the *Open Exercise* tape which she thought might prove "stronger." She felt occasional touches of pain, but not enough to cause her to wince.

When Eileen used the self-hypnosis suggestions without the tape she found they had little effect. In her own words, "It is my firm belief that Hemi-Sync is extremely effective during such surgery."

Another dental patient, Barbara, had been using Monroe tapes for two years when she decided for medical and cosmetic reasons to have her teeth straightened. This involved moving her teeth through bone by means of "corrective apparatus"—metal braces which would be needed for about two years. She was then thirty-three years old and was fortunate to find an orthodontist who would work with an adult; most prefer to work with children, when the procedure is much less troublesome.

Barbara was told that the process involved moving a tooth a fraction of an inch at a time and then allowing the bone to heal before moving it again. The emphasis on healing led her to think Hemi-Sync might help. She decided to use *Mission Night*, a music tape with sound signals embedded, *One Month Patterning*, as most appointments were at monthly intervals, and a Focus 12 tape for reinforcement. She also created her own affirmation which she used with each tape session.

In the early weeks of the treatment, Barbara felt a good deal of pain but this eventually receded. Both she and her dentist noted that progress was far more rapid than anticipated, and the procedure was completed in about half the predicted time.

A final example is Joy who, owing to fear of pain, had not allowed a dentist to look into her mouth for over fifteen years. Eventually the time came when she needed to have three cavities filled and ten old mercury fillings replaced. The night before treatment she played the *Pain Control* tape continuously while she slept and again on awakening. The dentist was curious and supportive of her decision not to have gas or injection and allowed her to listen to the tape while he worked.

"I was not overly confident that I would make it through unaided by anesthesia," she said, "but I was highly motivated to try. There was no discomfort as the dentist removed, redrilled, and cleaned out seven of the old fillings. Growing more confident, I signaled him to continue. The last three were deep, large cavities that he needed to redrill even deeper. He worked for one and a half hours to complete all the drilling. We took a break. I rose from the chair with thirteen gaping holes in my mouth, my body a little stiff from holding tension, but feeling great.

"Thinking the worst was over, I switched to a favorite popular music tape to enjoy while he filled the cavities, and was caught totally unaware by unexpected pain. In need of immediate relief, I used the number sequence suggestion from *Pain Control* instead of taking time to change tapes—and I was fine! What a pleasure to have completed the entire procedure in one visit, nearly free of pain, and feeling fine afterwards. I feel involved and part of the development of an extraordinary technology."

* * * * *

What emerges from these accounts is that the hemispheric synchronization process has been found by many individuals to be of major assistance in pain control and in overcoming fear or anxiety concerning dental work. Which particular tapes to use seems to be a matter of individual preference, but it appears that *Pre-Op, Pain Control*, and Metamusic tapes are likely to be helpful.

They Said It Was a Miracle: A Personal Story

Bill Tyler, age sixty, was employed as a driver for a major national delivery service. In June 1991, while driving, he lost consciousness owing to an escape of diesel fumes into the cab of his truck and crashed into a highway bridge abutment at about sixty miles per hour. The force of the impact ripped his seat from its anchorage and hurled him, still strapped in his seat, through the windshield. The truck was entirely demolished—it was not even identifiable as a truck after the accident. But Bill Tyler survived—no one knows how. The police and the emergency room doctor both described his survival as an unequivocal "miracle."

Mr. Tyler was taken to a nearby hospital, where it was determined that he had no broken bones or internal injuries. He had massive contusions—a reconstruction of the accident showed that his flight through the air had been stopped when he hit the concrete structure of the bridge—and many cuts from the shattered glass and metal. Just twenty-four hours after the accident he was sent home into his wife's care, where he spent the next four months recuperating.

Bill Tyler's daughter knew about Hemi-Sync and had used the tapes for herself. As soon as she heard about the accident she sent her father a package containing a battery-powered Walkman and four tapes: *Pain Control, Circulation, Brain: Repair & Maintenance,* and *Emergency: Injury.* For some hours after the accident, Bill's body felt completely numb, but as soon as feeling returned he began to experience very severe pain. His doctor had prescribed heavy doses of codeine. Bill is the type of person who in normal circumstances would not take even an aspirin, but he was glad to have the codeine at hand. However, it seemed to have little or no effect on the pain in his bones, joints and muscles, and although he was never one to complain he described this level of pain as excruciating. He was unable to lie down in any comfortable position or to sleep for more than a few moments at a time, and he could not walk at all.

Bill's daughter urged him to listen to *Pain Control* as soon as it arrived. She says, "It's a measure of how much pain he was in that he was agreeable to listen to a cassette tape in an effort to alleviate it—he is a very pragmatic, rather old-fashioned man who normally would be extremely reluctant to try anything so radical!" But the results were dramatic. He was able to reach a semi-trance state almost immediately, and although he reported that he was aware of the pain he was able to view it with detachment, as if he were outside himself. He listened to *Pain Control* and the other tapes over and over again, lying for hours at a time in a "suspended" state and getting significant rest with occasional deep sleep. His body began to heal rapidly, and within a few days most of his stitches could be removed. The headaches from the concussion he sustained subsided quickly with the use of the *Brain Repair* tape, and within two weeks there was marked improvement in his ability to think and speak clearly.

When Mr.Tyler began walking again he found much discomfort in one ankle. An x-ray one month after the accident revealed a previously unidentified fracture. The doctor who examined him put the leg in an air cast and advised him to keep his weight off it for another two or three weeks but was astounded at the rapidity with which the bones healed and in perfect alignment as if they had been in splints. Had the tapes helped this to happen, as his daughter believes?

When fully recovered, Mr Tyler returned the tapes to his daughter. Although, as she says, he is newly impressed with the awe-inspiring powers of the mind, he has no immediate desire to explore this area further. He returned to work in October, a few short months after an accident that would have killed most people. His physical health was not quite as robust as it was before the accident, but he is making progress daily. His daughter firmly believes the tapes have long-lasting residual effects, and are continuing to help in his recovery.

Applications: Mind

Chapter 4
Education and Training

In a paper written in 1984, Professor Devon Edrington commented that, while research into the nature of human consciousness in the last half-century had yielded remarkable insights, it was scandalous that educators had largely ignored their pedagogical significance. To illustrate his argument, he quoted from the late Brendan O'Regan, of the Institute of Noetic Sciences:

> Over the past couple of decades, in a wide variety of fields, numerous techniques and methods have been quietly devised, applied and tested—techniques that at the very least promise to give the population at large significantly increased access to their own potentials and capacities. The puzzle remains: why are we not applying these techniques more extensively, and how does it happen that the mainstream educational institutions have largely ignored even the most conservative pieces of information regarding these matters?

The last ten years have seen little, if any, progress in this area. Educational bureaucracies, as Robert Sornson points out below, are wary of innovation and suspicious of change. Hence it is mainly those teachers whose circumstances allow them a measure of individual freedom and who are themselves open-minded who are able to apply these new techniques. Edrington himself was one of these; another was JoDee Owens, a Tacoma Public Schools teacher, whose use of specially designed Hemi-Sync tapes played through loudspeakers with first-grade classes resulted, according to an independent evaluation, in "a great deal of independence and cooperation on the part of her class."

More recently, two small-scale trials in Cambridge, England, have produced promising results. In one, Metamusic was used with three creative writing classes whose ages ranged from eleven to sixteen. The Head of English Studies reported: "All the students experienced a detachment from the perceived experience. This detachment was contrasted with a sense of involvement which came out in metaphor and transitions built upon each other to a higher degree than usual in creative writing classes. This contrast between a phase of mental detachment and one of free imaginative involvement was one of the most interesting aspects of the experiment."

The second trial was organized by the Russell Centre for a small group of seventeen-year-olds preparing for their examinations to determine entry to university. These students claimed to suffer from "examination nerves" which, they felt, sapped their confidence and affected their performance. Four sessions using H-PLUS exercises were sufficient to enable them to relax at will and achieve belief in themselves; the examinations, involving some twenty-seven hours of written and practical work, proved trouble-free and all obtained the grades they desired.

This chapter contains accounts of the use of Hemi-Sync in five very different educational situations. Robert Sornson, a senior administrator in special education, describes his work with children and introduces the Teen Tapes educational project; Barbara Bullard explains the many ways in which she uses Hemi-Sync tapes with her undergraduate classes; Mark Douglas comments on his workshops for traders in the Chicago stock and futures markets, and Dr.Raymond Waldkoetter provides a detailed account of his work with different groups of military students over the past ten years. Dr. Suzanne Morris describes her work with teachers concerned with rehabilitation and special education, blending intuitive and rational approaches. Finally, Professor Gregory Carroll discusses the ethical considerations surrounding the use of this technology in the classroom.

These are not the only ways in which Hemi-Sync is used in training situations. It has proved helpful with dyslexic children and those whose learning is affected by poor sight. In music and art education, it has been used to reduce student anxiety and then to aid concentration and stimulate creativity. Other areas in which the process has been introduced include management training and the rehabilitation of prison inmates. Improved ability to relax, better control of stress, heightened creativity, and more closely focused attention are among the observed effects.

Special Education
Robert Sornson, Ed.S.

Robert Sornson is Executive Director of Special Education for Northill Public Schools in Michigan. He has developed a set of twenty taped exercises, each carrying appropriate Hemi-Sync signals, now in use in special education departments in schools throughout the state. He is currently engaged in further research into the possible applications of Hemi-Sync for children with emotional problems. In July 1990, he introduced the Teen Tapes educational pilot project in an address to the Professional Division of The Monroe Institute, in which he also discussed the difficulties of introducing innovative projects into the public education system and described the effects of Hemi-Sync on young children with a variety of disabilities.

My prime interest is in the application of the Hemi-Sync process, in making it work for children, in helping to improve a system which needs improvement in many different ways. Public education at the moment is especially interesting; there are so many pressures for change, demands for change, and yet as an institution it's marvelously adapted to resist change. Hemi-Sync may, over time, help to overcome that resistance.

Today's public education has been bureaucratized so much that it is almost impossible to make the sweeping types of reforms that you might see in a corporate climate. In the private sector, someone can come in, work with the CEO, and change a corporate climate within two years. But in education there are enormous barriers to those kinds of change. Most change comes from the ground up in education. The practitioners are the ones who change the process; yet they exist within a form of bureaucracy that is replete with obstacles—legal, bureaucratic, and traditional—that prevent those changes. So if we are to make changes that could affect countless thousands of schoolchildren we need to work from the ground up.

We need to have products that work practically, easily, fairly simply, without much technical explanation. Interestingly, most people do not ask me anything beyond the rather cursory information I give them about how Hemi-Sync works. All they want to know is that if they put it in a tape recorder, will it make a difference to children. That saves me having to launch into a technical explanation.

I am often surprised at finding myself in education, where originally I had no intention of being. But I kept being pushed in that direction, the biggest push coming when, aged twenty-three, I was running an orchard in Michigan and was exposed to pesticides, the effect of which was that I suffered serious neurologic damage and nearly died. For some time I was in very bad shape, from which it took a very long time to recover. That experience changed my attitude radically; I became interested in neurology, chemistry, and bio-chemistry because now these areas were important to me. Hitherto things came easily to me; but now I could sympathize with people, children especially, with severe learning difficulties. I could share the experience of someone for whom things did not fit, memory did not function, balance was not there. Vestibular and hearing problems were related to my neurological condition. This change in viewpoint pushed me toward education.

So, although I was still largely impaired, I took my master's degree in special education—without opening a book as I could not then read—and found a job in that field. My first principal advised me to keep my class happy and not to work them too hard. How wrong he was! Experience showed me that most children in special education are no different from anyone else; they have incredible capacities. They are all different, with each mind working in its own unique way and, like all of us, each student perceives the world in his or her own way.

I am particularly interested in the neurology of thought process, and certainly how Hemi-Sync affects neurology. One advantage of being in special education is that no one comes in to see what you are doing in the classroom. Hence I could use Hemi-Sync tapes; I could bring in a recliner so that children could listen in comfort. I had freedom, and because of that I was able to learn so much about kids that would have been impossible in any other educational setting. Now that I am in special education administration I still have that freedom; I can introduce things into classes which otherwise would have to undergo a cumbersome review process through the whole hierarchy of boards and committees.

I first used Hemi-Sync in a classroom setting with a couple of boys labeled emotionally impaired who also showed signs of attention deficit disorder. They were hyperactive, always in trouble, involved in drug abuse, from very dysfunctional families—there were many reasons for their impairment. Previously I had been involved in work with children with cerebral palsy, using TENS machines which give a mild electrical stimulus to the brain and produce a gentle relaxation effect. I measured self-concept and learning during the same time, and found extraordinary changes in both over two months. It was then that I was introduced to Hemi-Sync, and I realized there was a possibility of achieving similar effects with much less difficulty and with a less invasive approach—and with less red tape—and so we tried it.

Everyone liked it, especially the children who were even prepared to fight for it! I recall especially David, one of the most extreme instances of learning deficiency I had come across. He began listening—he was not even sitting in a comfortable chair—and within a few moments he was out—and the exercise was "Retain, Recall, Release," not the most exciting or interesting tape in the world. He liked it, and so did his friend. One day I found them beginning to fight for whose turn it was to listen to the tape!

We tried with others and noted changes in attitude, comprehension, behavior, and levels of relaxation. I began to query what was happening when I observed that kids who listened to Hemi-Sync over no more than two or three weeks seemed to have lasting effects. Why would that be? I have some theories, but I still don't know the answer, although the ongoing research should eventually prove if my theories are correct.

I went on to try tapes with children with a variety of problems—learning deficiency, physical problems, cerebral palsy—and they had generally a positive effect. Most noticeable, however, was the positive effect on children whom I would describe as poorly cortically integrated—those who do not seem able to integrate information from one side of the cortex to the other. These are the children—many of them in special education—who move in a disjointed way, with one side not working well with the other. Many have problems with their eyes, which do not work well together; they do not seem able to focus clearly on a given object. These are types of underlying problems which cause the problems that we are aware of, and which often we ignore in seeking to diagnose or help the child. We concentrate on the basic skills, but these children may find these skills incredibly difficult to master, and by insisting on them we may do more harm than good and create a non-cooperative attitude as well. These underlying problems need to be dealt with, and it seems that Hemi-Sync helps to deal with the basic neurology, especially for those who are poorly integrated cortically.

Examples—and we may recognize some of these in ourselves—are children who can listen to language, understand the words and meanings, but not be aware of the tone of voice, not notice the inflection or the pattern of language, not notice the body language and be able to put it together with the words. They take things literally, do not understand humor, irony, puns; they are typically those who are not putting information together properly from one side of the cortex to the other. Language, as it deals with symbols, is essentially a left-brain function, while pattern-recognition is a function of the right brain, including intuitive pattern-recognition, an important part of learning for so many of us. These are children who can do a rote-math problem—addition, multiplication, etc.—but cannot put it together with the concept underlying the problem. They can do division on paper, but in the context of a story or everyday life they are lost. They do not see what it means; they cannot connect the pattern with the specific rote information. This is poor cortical integration. Good learning is whole-brain learning; good communication is whole-brain communication. Good mathematics involves spatial and pattern recognition together with good memory and symbolic use. Every aspect of learning that works well involves both sides of the brain; so cortical integration is especially important.

There are many different ways to get children to integrate cortically. There are physical methods: encouraging young children to crawl and to use their hands, moving them from one visual field to another; gross motor activities; exercises using agility, using one arm then the other, swinging, running, playing—what most children do very naturally.

Cortical integration closely connects with sensory integration—an expression that in educational circles is still largely taboo. Sensory integration is more than just crossing the hemispheres at the cortex; it is integration at every level within the brain. And sensory integration is affected by Hemi-Sync—the child who suddenly sits up and starts to look around and makes that eye contact for the very first time. Instead of being overloaded sensorially, the brain seems to calm down, the level of arousal drops in some—or increases in others—and the world becomes something the child can deal with.

I have had the good fortune to work with autistic children, who provide the best opportunity to study sensory integration. These children are overwhelmed by sensory information; they come into a room, and the lights, the sounds, the background noises, and the people overwhelm them. They try to block it all out, and they perform all kinds of strange activities to do so. They start flapping, rocking, squealing, running around on tip-toe, tightening their shoulders. Yet many of them are extremely bright in many ways. I know one seven-year-old who can solve any kind of math problem immediately, and another child who remembers every single thing that occurred in his life, and another who remembers any amount of data yet who cannot apply that data. These children show the greatest deficiency in sensory integration that can be manifested. Many people will tell you that autistic children will never be helped, that their condition is irreversible, and progress is impossible. But it does not always have to be that way.

When I first started to work with these youngsters I wanted to use more than Hemi-Sync. I wanted to use motor programs where they would be doing lots of movement to get their brains working and organizing. What you stimulate, grows; think of the thousands of neurological connections that take place in the smallest instant, the neurological changes that are constantly happening, which give you the capacity, the framework, for new types of transferred information. This is what autistic children need.

Let me take Jacob as an example. He was seven when I first saw him, extremely autistic and also very bright. His parents desperately wanted him to have as normal a life as possible, yet he was not a normal child by a very long way. As an administrator I was called in to look at the situation and I found that Jacob was behaving extremely disruptively in his first-grade classroom. The school was trying to keep him in the mainstream, instead of placing him with severely retarded autistic children. They wanted to find some way in which he could grow, develop, change, mature—some way through which he would not be destined to become just one among the others. We began with a good motor program and some Hemi-Sync. The first time we used Hemi-Sync he turned and looked at the aide who was overseeing him (who would carry him out if he became too disruptive) and established eye contact for the very first time.

A week later he was out for a walk. It was early October in Michigan. He looked around and said, "The leaves are falling—it must be autumn." This was the first time he had ever noticed anything like that. The next week he was looking out of his classroom window; he turned to his aide and shouted, "There's a pine tree out there!" He had been looking out of that window for months but was so sensorially disorganized that he had not been aware there was a pine tree there—he had never registered it. That is the level of disorganization with which some of these children have to live. Now I can tell you that Jacob is going into third grade and I could, if necessary, pull away all the support he has and leave him in third grade, and he would do well. In a year or so the only noticeable difference between Jacob and the rest of his class will be that he's extremely bright with an IQ near 150.

Hemi-Sync is not a magic bullet for children like Jacob. It does not organize his neurology. But it does something that allows his own brain, his own mind, his own spirit to organize itself in a different way so that he can start to go out and get the experiences he needs; to see pine trees, to move in a more coordinated fashion without all that weird behavior, to relax in such a way that he can learn socially and academically, learn as a human being.

All the cortical information is passed from one side of the cortex to the other through that little band of tissue about the size of your little finger, the corpus callosum. I feel that when we are using Hemi-Sync of any kind in some way the brain is starting to communicate with itself better. By improving this communication across the corpus callosum we are stimulating nerve use and when you stimulate a brain cell it grows and develops. I can easily prove that things are happening to connect the right and left cortical hemispheres, and because children become more sensorially integrated I assume that connection is also happening at another level between the cortex and the lower portions of the brain. Now I am awaiting the research that will show us pictures of this happening and will tell us what is happening in terms of the neurochemistry, what changes are occurring in the neuropeptides, and in the electromagnetic fields that exist in and around the brain and which are important in brain function but which we do not often take into account because they are so difficult to measure.

The Teen Tapes are a special project of mine which I have scripted to deal with issues that are important to teenagers. There are twenty in all, divided into four sets of five. In the first set we look at issues related to self-concept and self-esteem, prefaced by a different type of relaxation, to teach children how to relax their bodies, helped by Hemi-Sync. Once they are deeply relaxed we move into introducing them to specific tools and showing them specific ways in which they can act to help them defend their self-concept and build their self-esteem and learn to relate to others in a positive way. When you feel good about yourself you are far more likely to be happy and fulfilled both in school and in life altogether.

The second set deals with school improvement—the whole process of being successful in studies. The third set deals with decision-making skills, goal-setting, solutions. Dealing with family and personal solutions is vitally important for teenagers—I wish that I had learned this years ago. Teenagers these days have to make decisions that the older generation never dreamed about; decisions about drugs and sex in junior high school and even in elementary school, relating to peer pressure of a new and intense kind. They need skills to help them in these difficult situations, skills that unfortunately they have very few opportunities to acquire.

The last set of five deals with creativity and harmony. I feel that ideally students should listen to a set of tapes three or four times and then go on to the next set, spending about a month on each set.

We have used these tapes in a variety of settings. For example, we used the Teen Tapes with two students in a day treatment program. This program is a consequence of the policy of returning mentally ill people to the community instead of keeping them in institutions. These two were severely mentally ill, but they like Hemi-Sync, they are maintaining, and they have not had to return to the institution. In contrast, a student who became blind at fourteen is using the tapes and reckons they are proving of enormous help to him. A fourteen-year-old girl who has been in and out of mental hospitals for years has responded extremely positively; for the first time she has been able to recognize when things were beginning to go wrong and has been able to ask for her medication and for help and support. They have also been used by a group of athletes, with excellent positive response, and pilot schemes are in progress or being organized in many areas.

To extend the use of the Teen Tapes we need to consider the obstacles. People in education generally have little experience of this sort of approach and we have to deal with school boards and other bodies not known for their imagination. Solutions are needed here. We also need to investigate new products incorporating Hemi-Sync and to research how to market them. Learning-disabled children, autistic children, the cortically poorly integrated, the hyperkinetic— and not forgetting the would-be successful athletes—there are a lot of children who need a lot of help, who are crying out for help. Proper application of Hemi-Sync technology can provide many of these children with help along the way.

Language Learning and Superlearning
Barbara Bullard, M.A.

Barbara Bullard (see also Chapter 2) is a professor of Speech Communication in California and has been teaching in the areas of language and communication for over twenty-five years. She is listed in Outstanding Educators of America, 1974 *and* Outstanding Scholars in Community Colleges, 1987-88.

For more than ten years a major topic in my lectures has been the importance of bilateral synchronized brain waves in superlearning—a super performance learning state. I have also recognized that this brain state is a significant factor in eliciting the "trophotropic response," the autonomic healing mechanism of the body. Over the years I had collected a number of audio tapes that claimed to produce this synchronized brain pattern but, I discovered, failed to do so. Many of the tapes I tried did, in one way or another, facilitate learning, but none of them was effective in promoting or aiding self-healing.

When, four years ago, I heard of the H-PLUS series I decided I might as well try those and I took the list of tapes into the under-graduate class I was teaching—the subject was Intrapersonal Com-munications. We selected thirty-two tapes to be divided between the eighteen members of the class.

I was pleasantly surprised by the positive impact of the tapes as reported by the students within two weeks of use. Among the benefits reported were overcoming learning blocks, accelerated learning, easy weight loss, getting rid of negative or painful memories, changing negative attitudes toward situations or other people, and giving up smoking. I was asked to order more tapes and we sent off for another seventy-six. Students reported further chan-ges in their own attitudes and behavior and in their self-healing ability.

Following these impressive results, I attended a Gateway program. The computer-generated topographic brain maps illustrating hemispheric synchronization convinced me that what hitherto I believed was happening was happening in fact.

I have continued to extend the use of the tapes with my students. Initially my interest focused on helping them with their learning skills, their ability to concentrate and to deal with test and math anxiety. On entering the college many of them need to improve their study habits and learning skills before they can begin to make other progress. At least fifty students have used the PAL (Progressive Accelerated Learning) album to help with their concentration levels and their retention. Many of them find it helpful to play the *Concentration* tape quietly while they study, using headphones if they need to eliminate outside noise. Most of them find the *Retain-Recall-Release* exercise useful in preparing for tests, and they reckon these two tapes have helped them raise their scores a minimum of one grade. Other tapes that have proved helpful include H-PLUS exercises *Imprint* (for memory) and *Think Fast* (for creative thinking, comprehension, and speedier understanding). Nearly thirty students have used *Buy the Numbers* to help them pass math and understand its principles in their pursuit of the Associate of Arts degree. The *Attention* exercise helps them to settle down to study; *Options* may spark creativity; *Speak Up* aids in overcoming nervousness about speaking out in class or in public, and *Make Your Day* is useful in encouraging them to make effective use of each day and to overcome procrastination.

A favorite tape with students is *Catnapper,* which provides the benefit of a full sleep cycle in a thirty-minute nap. This helps in overcoming the tiredness of final exam week and the aftereffects of cramming. Many students who work full-time use this exercise for stress release and to compensate for lost sleep. Some, together with members of their families, have found *Eat/No Eat* and *Nutricia* useful in controlling eating habits and weight loss (they helped me lose twenty pounds and then to maintain my weight). They have also helped with those suffering from anorexia and bulimia—not uncommon conditions among students.

Of the exercises useful in overcoming negative memories and emotions, *Off-Loading* seemed the most effective. This is purported to help release "restrictive and destructive mental, emotional and physical patterns which impede achievement of your needs and goals." I have witnessed that this tape helps in the release of memories of abuse, rape, hurt, and disappointment. One forty-year-old student used it to assist in overcoming a strong irritation with her husband's behavior—and also to lose twenty pounds in weight. It worked so well that three weeks later she started using it to stop drinking and smoking. She achieved all these goals within six weeks, certain that the tape helped her to overcome the inertia and fear associated with these problems. Other students have used *Off-Loading* for weight loss, stopping abuse of drugs and alcohol, and "mending broken hearts."

A major area in which I have found the tapes to be especially effective is in aiding the healing process. One of the first occasions when I suggested this was for a student with AIDS. He came to me distressed at his declining T cell count. We chose the H-PLUS exercise *Regenerate,* with the thought that it would assist him in visualizing the production of new T cells. Three weeks later he was tested again and his T cell count had doubled. His doctor asked if he had any idea what might account for this significant increase and my student told him about *Regenerate.* Two weeks later a similar gain was recorded. The student obtained four more tapes for friends of his with AIDS, and they too experienced comparable increases in T cell counts. Since then I have recommended this tape to four other HIV-positive patients to help rebuild their immune systems—again, similar results are reported.

It seems that the immune system may also respond to the H-PLUS exercises *Tune Up* and *Restorative Sleep;* both have been helpful with long-term disabilities and post-operative recovery. For specific problems the tapes focusing on the lungs, brain, and heart have proved valuable. The *Lungs* exercise works well for those with AIDS-related pneumonia and is used in two HIV-Positive Immunity Programs. The *Heart: Repair & Maintenance* tape I used myself for a prolapsed valve problem, and I have also suggested it for several students who were being treated for panic attack disorder.

Another useful exercise is *Circulation.* For five years I suffered from edema in my left foot, which failed to respond to treatment. However, when I first tried this function the swelling reduced almost immediately and now, after frequent use over the past three years, it seldom swells at all. This exercise also relieved a lifetime problem of unnaturally cold hands and feet, which meant that I had to sleep under a heavy weight of blankets. Within two months of using the tape this condition ceased to trouble me. The *Circulation* tape helped too with migraine headaches. My belief is that by redistributing blood throughout the body in a balanced manner it enables the engorged blood in the head to dissipate.

After a year of recommending the taped exercises to students I was asked to talk about them in public. This brought me into contact with older people, many of whom were especially interested in the tapes dealing with sight and hearing. The *Sensory: Hearing* tape proved valuable with cases of tinnitus, while more than thirty people used the *Sensory: Seeing* exercise with much success. One noteworthy case is that of an eighty-year-old nun, due for a cataract operation. Her doctors feared the herpes infection in her eyes might flare up and perhaps lead to blindness, but she insisted on going through with the operation, given added confidence through using the tape. The operation was successful, with no complications. She continued with the tape afterwards and greatly surprised her doctor by the virtually total recovery of her vision. When she told him about the tape he replied, "Whatever it was, it worked!"

I am convinced by my experience over four years that the H-PLUS tapes are effective in a number of ways, including improving memory, concentration, goal facilitation, weight loss, and various healing effects. I have found the tapes to be valuable tools for learning and growth that accord easily with any individual philosophy. My students and friends are enthusiastically encouraged to try them at least once, because personal experience, here as elsewhere, is the best teacher.

Developing Winning Attitudes:
Traders, Trading and Hemi-Sync
Mark Douglas

Mark Douglas is president of Trading Behavior Dynamics, Inc., *a Chicago-based consulting firm that works with individual traders, certified trading advisers, banks, and brokerage firms internationally. His book* The Disciplined Trader: Developing Winning Attitudes *has sold widely, especially in the trading community.*

As a natural outgrowth of my book, which deals with the psychology of trading both the stock and futures markets, I developed an intensive two-day workshop, "How to Become a Disciplined Trader." This workshop focuses on helping traders understand and develop the mental framework necessary to interact with the market environment in the most effective ways. H-PLUS is an essential component of the workshop.

The workshop's basic premise is that there are many beliefs, common or culturally learned, that prevent people from becoming consistently successful as traders. The generally accepted industry statistic is that less than two percent of traders achieve any measure of consistency. The other ninety-eight percent either consistently lose, or they can produce consistent earnings up to some internally imposed limit, after which they unconsciously sabotage their success, lose their earnings, and begin the cycle again.

Consistent success is possible. Yet it is an unavoidable fact of trading that, regardless of how good a trader becomes at analyzing and predicting market behavior, he will at times inevitably be wrong and lose money. But the typical trader is unwilling to accept this inevitability and, in the process of trying to avoid it, actually creates the very experiences he fears.

When one considers that we all have within us the natural propensity to avoid pain, physically and emotionally, it is easy to see how traders get themselves into trouble. Among the mass beliefs of our culture is the tacit agreement that losing money and being wrong are intrinsically pain-producing. As the trader attempts to avoid those conditions, he ignores, distorts, or rationalizes information that indicates he is in a losing trade. So, rather than acknowledging that reality and cutting his losses, he maintains his position until the pain of losing one more dollar is greater than the fear of admitting he is wrong.

Many traders achieve consistent earnings after attending one of my workshops. However, to do this the trader must first recognize that the market environment is in almost every way different from the cultural environment in which he was brought up. He must then learn to alter or neutralize the very fundamental beliefs and fears that were learned before he decided to become a trader.

In the workshop, traders learn mental techniques to monitor their thoughts or "states of being" to determine if they are in states that are most conducive to giving themselves money, or at least not giving their money away. They learn to identify the beliefs out of which they are operating any given moment and to determine if these beliefs are appropriate to their goal of becoming consistently successful traders. For instance, a trader must be able to perceive being wrong and losing money as conditions offering information rather than as conditions producing pain. If the trader assesses that a particular belief is dysfunctional and he completely understands why it won't work, he then uses the "Plus—No More, No More" Function Command from the H-PLUS *De-Hab* tape to neutralize it.

This Hemi-Sync tape is valuable because it provokes a very active response to a very specific issue, and I have found when working with mental energy the more specific one is the better the results. Once the Function Command is installed, the trader must learn when, where, and how to use it. Hence I provide specific instructions for activating the Function Command consciously and appropriately. Assuming the trader has learned to recognize when he is operating out of a belief inconsistent with his goals, at the moment he realizes this he must capture whatever thought or emotion is being experienced and make it tangible. Traders are taught to do this by either stating the thought or emotion as a belief or by using some form of mental imagery to give the beliefs as much substance as possible. Once they are completely clear about what they want to release, they state the Command with as much conviction as possible—"Plus—No More, No More!" The greater the energy behind the conviction, the more pronounced a shift they will feel.

Other than the effects produced by the low-frequency binaural beat stimulation, it is the high level of participation required—mental focus, personal choice, and willingness to use the Function Command—that makes the H-PLUS system so effective in helping people create desired change.

About a month after the workshop I send survey forms to participants asking them to indicate on a scale from one to ten (1) their ability to identify and capture beliefs, (2) the strength of their convictions when they use the Command, and (3) the effectiveness of the Command in neutralizing beliefs. Replies indicate a very strong correlation between the participants' perceived abilities to identify exactly what beliefs they want to neutralize, the strength of their convictions, and the effectiveness rating they assign to the Function Command.

Interestingly, most people who take the workshop have had very little exposure to information or concepts related to self-awareness or learning to change oneself through directed conscious effort. Despite this, virtually everyone's initial reaction to H-PLUS is overwhelmingly positive, regardless of how skeptical or uncomfortable they may have been at first listening.

It is clear that the system resonates with people at a very deep and fundamental level, regardless of whether they understand the dynamics at work.

Military Training and Development
Raymond O. Waldkoetter, Ed.D.

Dr. Ray Waldkoetter is a personnel management analyst who has been involved in promoting organizational efficiency and performance-enhancement techniques for the U.S. Army. He is also a psychologist in private practice. In recent years he has conducted several training studies using the Hemi-Sync technology in the areas of stress reduction, counseling, and language learning, among others.

Consciousness-altering brain-wave entrainment, occurring directly from known sound pulse stimulation, allows adjustment of attention or concentration to experience whatever state is most compatible with particular awareness and purpose. It seems reasonable, therefore, that education and training can utilize various Hemi-Sync procedures, and in the following pages I shall describe some of the intensive experiences in military training programs which have demonstrated positive results using this technology. These experiences help to illustrate how military students may react to the use of sound-wave patterns in their training, and how these patterns may be adapted to enhance competent instruction and treatment. At the same time, it must be recognized that there is probably no technology that will improve inadequate training programs and instruction.

In late 1982, an Army study was conducted using an enlisted radio/television broadcasting class in the Department of Defense Information School at Fort Benjamin Harrison, Indiana, with the aim of reducing stress to enhance learning. From 1983 onwards, Hemi-Sync tapes have been used in support of counseling with ongoing student problems, both personal and academic. In 1984 a foreign language program to provide refresher training for soldiers who might be needed for special missions overseas was initiated. This training was based partly on the belief that learning is improved in a more relaxed mental state with lessened tension, and this program is still producing superior language performance. In October 1990, a study commenced in the Defense Information School to find out if use of a Progressive Accelerated Learning album of taped exercises would show identifiable learning improvements and how use of this album might contribute to the training program for a group of officers and civilians in the Public Affairs Course. Additionally, since 1978 the Hemi-Sync process has been used with several military and civilian personnel in a wide variety of employment and personal advisory needs. At this level, the tapes have shown the potential to change to desired behaviors, increase learning ability, improve sleep patterns, and reduce pain responses.

These studies and experiences will be discussed in a scientific context to represent the possibilities of the use of this technology without suggesting that it makes extravagant claims. It is, however, clear that its use is worthwhile in relation to course training, school counseling, language learning, psychological consulting, and advanced military training.

Audio-Guided Stress Reduction

For this project, a training program was devised with The Monroe Institute of eight taped exercises for use with a stereo cassette player. The test unit selected was the basic broadcaster's course (BBC) for lower-ranked enlisted personnel of the Defense Information School. The broadcaster's training involves conditions of time pressure and high skill requirements and could be favorably affected by technology which reduces stress. A trial demonstration was experienced by a number of the staff and faculty to assure the absence of risk and the promotion of relaxation.

The technology was made available to the test class of twenty-two students for ten weeks, covering the Voice and Diction, Radio, and Television training segments. Two control groups were arranged for course performance and stress responses. The exercises covered an introduction to the process, relaxation, attention, concentration, sleep, peak performance and specific performance instructions. The schedule involved use of the tapes both during the day and after class and at weekends, with the use diminishing as the course progressed. While all the students met the basic selection requirements for their training, this class was slightly atypical in that several students had initial academic deficiencies (67 percent deficiency status compared with 54 percent for the course performance control group). Hence a slightly lower overall class performance might be expected.

The effects of the technology were to be measured in relation to performance and relaxation. Students were observed periodically during training, and five questionnaires were completed during the course, with four more, covering stress and course experiences, use of the tapes, peer/classmate opinions, and instructor observations, administered at the end. Attrition during the course reduced the numbers graduating to nine; this, though quite heavy, was not exceptional where exacting broadcasting performance standards had to be met. The test class was compared to three immediately graduated classes for course performance and to the immediately prior graduated class (of ten students) for stress control.

Five designated test objectives were measured by collecting questionnaire data designed to probe objective and subjective experiences related to the tape use and responses. Course performance records were also analyzed to compare any actual differences between classes which might be related to the use of the technology.

The first objective was to evaluate the acceptability of Hemi-Sync by enlisted students. The average (mean) rating on all the following sixteen behavioral characteristics showed moderate or high improvement with tape use. It was to be expected by chance that eight of these characteristics would show little or no improvement if students found Hemi-Sync unacceptable.

> More energy available
> Fewer "down" periods
> More restful sleep
> Less need for coffee, alcohol, etc.
> Feel more healthy
> Improved self-control
> Improved study habits
> Less irritability/frustration
> Improved reaction to physical activity
> Increased alertness
> Improved concentration
> Improved fluency
> Improved retention of information
> Improved ability to think clearly
> More relaxed
> Less tension

This finding was statistically significant as it would be likely to occur only one time out of a hundred by chance in such a group.

Nearly 89 percent of the graduating test students rated the radio-performance tape as "helpful" to "very helpful." This is statistically significant, occurring only five times out of a hundred by chance for such a group. Eighty-nine percent of these students also described the tapes of being of some degree of help during their completion of course requirements.

Eighty-two percent of the initial test students claimed the tapes had helped to improve their performance in the first week of training, another statistically significant finding, while 72 percent of the graduating students responded with positive comments in a post-test interview supporting the use of the technology.

The second objective was to have the faculty evaluate the acceptability of Hemi-Sync use by students. The faculty members observed that the technology was at least as successful as their usual procedures and could help toward the needed stress-reduction. They saw no impairing results and regarded the technology as an acceptable instructional approach.

The third objective was to evaluate the need to adapt the Hemi-Sync technology for use in the course. None of the tapes was rated "not helpful" by the class; the range of ratings was from "barely helpful" to "very helpful." This indicated that some tapes might benefit from revision of sound quality or content. Students would have preferred more time for Hemi-Sync training during the course, with some editing of voice-over instruction.

The fourth objective was to evaluate the need to adapt performance measures in the course to provide tests of effectiveness of the Hemi-Sync technology. As no appropriate procedures existed, particular measuring considerations needed to be made, and five questionnaires were devised to collect data regarding Hemi-Sync and a screening procedure was designed to analyze course records and tests for objective data.

The fifth objective was to evaluate the effectiveness of the technology in training students on this course. The test class graduated 50 percent of its students, while the performance control group graduated 46 percent. Graduates for both classes were reduced to half or less of the initial groups by academic and administrative attrition, which could not be significantly reduced because the performance requirements emphasized in part individual aptitudes (voice quality, poise, etc.) rather than immediately trained skills. The difference between percentages graduating was not statistically significant but satisfied the school commanders with a practical budget-saving for the few additional graduates.

Test students generally displayed a distinctive number of positive training differences, which were favorable over the stress control group, toward their Hemi-Sync experiences, and over the performance control group in terms of enhanced stress reactions and performance responses. All the test students rated "performing practical exercises" as relaxing, compared to none in the stress control group; test students also rated improved behavioral characteristics and exceeded the performance control group in a number of ways.

As a result of this study, even though it was not wholly conclusive, further utilization of Hemi-Sync can be recommended in the area of accelerated training. In the small sample test, data was obtained in support of stress reduction and enhanced training performance, and it would appear that students could expect accelerated experiences through improved relaxation, favorable changes in actual performance or enhanced motivation. A more successful application of the technology would occur if the tapes and performance measures were precisely adapted to support the given training objectives. This evaluation suggested that where student performance met or exceeded standards, the technology would serve to induce relaxation and lessen the degree of task stress—less effort and more efficient work.

Both students and faculty members suggested Hemi-Sync technology would make an alternative counseling strategy for rapid acquisition training when training plans could not fully incorporate it in the regular schedule. If several students per class were retained with the help of this technology during one year, a tangible cost reduction would result.

Student Counseling

The work with the Broadcasting Course impressed some of the faculty members and administrative heads and led to the introduction of Hemi-Sync materials into an academic counseling program. Students with academic problems were casually referred to the tapes used in the BBC study with the simple explanation that these tapes were known to have helped some students reduce stress and improve concentration. Most of these students were repeating some part of the course and needed little direction on how to use the tapes. Their comments indicated that the tapes helped them sleep, study, prepare for class more efficiently, control nervousness, organize activities better, and retain greater information. Since 1983, more than 200 students have been counseled in this way and it appears that the tapes have not only helped these students academically and emotionally but have also protected the school's financial investment by graduating 200-plus students during that time.

On occasion, staff members borrowed tapes for themselves. Two examples may be cited. In the first, a young non-commissioned lady used the album of tapes created for the BBC course and scored so highly on a promotion evaluation test that her integrity was first questioned. Later she was promoted and commended for her outstanding achievement. In the second, a male NCO used the same tapes to help him in a competitive professional course and graduated in the top five percent. He freely attributed his success to the tapes' effect and was amazed at his level of concentration and the sense of time passing quickly.

No other attempts to facilitate academic achievement have approached this degree of consistently favorable response nor prevailed through the continuing pressure of school exigencies. Time and again, students using Hemi-Sync have shown increased awareness of their own needs and how better to organize their academic and related-life activities. One major result of Hemi-Sync exposure is the balancing of the individual's sense of awareness and coherence of reality. Awareness and reality are focused inwardly in a more functional pattern and immediately related to the external conditions for desired activity. Students seem to be able to perform more efficiently and be less distracted. Following from this state of improved mental and emotional equilibrium, students seem to do better on cognitive and multisensory tasks. Other students not participating in tape use or counseling have commented on how the tape exposure has helped those who were using them both in classroom performance and in emotional stability.

Language Training

In 1984, two young female teachers began a language training program at a western U.S. Army site designed to bring "refresher" material to specially trained combat-oriented soldiers, with the emphasis on the conversational use of the chosen language(s). The teachers combined the Georgy Lozanov teaching method with the use of music carrying embedded in it appropriate phased-sound signals. Both teachers were excellent language instructors who used selected text materials and unobtrusively presented the Hemi-Sync and music as a minor innovation.

Working with such disciplined and motivated students, the teachers expected accelerated learning and the speedy attainment of language proficiency. The added sounds enhanced the learning environment, and the teachers observed that the learning process was changing in a subtle but noticeable way. As the students followed directions, the teachers became aware that the atmosphere in class was relaxing and the students became more spontaneous in responding to teacher cues and questions. Enthusiasm was evident in the way class schedules were met and assignments were quickly accomplished. The Hemi-Sync signals and music were creating an environment where the students could concentrate better and without undue tension. Students later reported that they considered their language training as one of their most rewarding military experiences.

What seemed to occur in the classroom was a creative and valuable synthesis; even the teachers were not fully aware of the process as it happened for them and their students. As in the counseling program, there were therapeutic effects which helped to maintain the students' motivation and suspend any restraint in their personal learning styles and perception. With some variations in staffing and other support, this language training venture has been highly productive from its unheralded start in 1984, and for the value received it has been inexpensive training operated on a minimal budget. A more visionary military supervisor might have found a way to extend this program to other sites, but it remains an active source of highly successful language renewal. However, another study was conducted at a traditional U.S. Army language school where the Hemi-Sync technology was introduced into the curriculum without any noticeable effects. This was due to the rigidity of the traditional approach which failed to investigate in any depth what potential Hemi-Sync does have.

It is worth adding that one of the best reasons for recommending the Hemi-Sync plus music background as an adjunct to language training is the subtle effect on the teachers themselves. They derive most of the same benefits as the students but are able to crystallize their role as source and channel of information over and beyond the basic language material. Teachers—in any discipline—may rise to levels of awareness where they unconsciously utilize supranormal knowledge and guidance to enhance student behavior.

Auditory Guidance in Officer-Level Training

A further test of the value of Hemi-Sync in training was carried out with the Public Affairs Officer Course (PAOC) at the Defense Information School. The public affairs officers' training and job involve various pressures and skill demands across military community relations, public affairs communication and media, and broadcasting, and could be affected favorably by technology that reduces stress and enhances learning. Three test objectives were to be evaluated:

1. Determine if the Hemi-Sync process increases and augments subject-matter learning;

2. Determine if other learning experiences are positively affected by the use of the process; and

3. Determine if other positive behavioral experiences are activated by the process.

Test scores, training exercises, and related measures would provide the necessary evidence.

The trial ran for ten weeks in the fall of 1990. The PAOC class of forty-four officer and civilian students was divided into a test and a control group, with the test group using the Progressive Accelerated Learning album of six taped exercises. Instructions for tape use and a tape usage schedule were issued.

With the first objective, the test class did slightly better than its two predecessors, although not sufficiently so to be able to attribute the difference to the use of the tapes. However, on each of the four subject-matter tests on the major areas during the course, the test group exceeded the control group. Three-quarters of the students reported that they felt the tapes helped them generally in most if not all the subject areas.

The second objective findings showed that other learning experiences were positively affected to some degree by the Hemi-Sync process. Seven out of nine course task performances were indicated by majority ratings as improved by using the process, with "memorizing," "studying," and "taking tests" most favorably affected.

The third objective determined that other positive behavioral experiences were activated by the process. Four out of the six tapes were assessed by the majority as helpful, with *Concentration* and *Catnapper* most decidedly so.

Twenty-five percent of the students reported that they experienced unusual mental and/or physical changes during tape use, and it is operationally significant that students can experience unusual changes that are personally inspiring. In discussion, many students declared that the tapes gave them the sensation of being able to do more in less time and to organize assignments more efficiently. Improved study effort and relaxation appeared to occur with the test group.

To summarize, the Hemi-Sync tapes fulfilled several academic and personal needs as students progressed through their training, and those students with stated interest or need appeared to benefit most. Those who volunteered to take part merely out of curiosity may have profited only by an accidental foray into some aspect of altered consciousness. It is recommended that when feasible the tapes be used in a training context with added emphasis on counseling or self-development coaching to make individual and course objectives fully complementary. It is likely that the tapes would prove most valuable in training when used in a self-development counseling process.

This exploratory work verifies the utility of Hemi-Sync in relatively stressful group training programs, but the instructional and therapeutic value of the technology goes beyond adapting it to produce reliable group experiences. Although certain common group experiences may be planned and achieved, the ultimate value of the process lies in training each individual to develop his or her awareness to enhance performance, thereby enabling each to contribute to the group's greater creativity and capability.

Note: The views expressed in this article are those of the author and do not necessarily reflect positions by the U.S. Department of Defense or Department of the Army. Special thanks are due to Mrs. Patricia Russell for help in coordinating and presenting this material.

Recapturing the Intuitive in Therapy and Education

Suzanne Evans Morris, Ph.D.

Dr. Suzanne Morris is a speech-language pathologist, known internationally on account of her work with infants and young children. She organizes workshops and courses for children and their families and for professionals in the field, at her center near Charlottesville, Virginia. Here she discusses her recent work in adult continuing education.

My adult continuing education workshops are taught primarily to professionals working in the field of rehabilitation and special education. They last for five to seven days with between twenty and twenty-six participants; in the past seven years they have been attended by 467 therapists in total. The Hemi-Sync technology has been an integral part of the program since its inception, with Metamusic, the *Concentration* tape, and other music with appropriate signals embedded employed as a background for learning.

In the first four years of the program, a question asking for specific evaluation of participants' response to the Hemi-Sync music background was included on the evaluation form. Almost all participants (96 percent) indicated that with this music they felt more relaxed and more attentive than at other workshops. In a follow-up questionnaire four months after the workshop, approximately half of those responding said they were using Metamusic tapes in their therapy with children and adults.

An interesting trend emerged in the open-ended questions on the follow-up. Many participants said they felt more intuitive and connected with their clients since the workshop. However, they added that they were not fully comfortable with this since they did not know whether to trust the increased number of "hunches" that were emerging, nor did they know how to put this together with the more rational approach they had been taught. From this feedback, a new workshop, focusing on the issues of intuition and the blending of intuitive and rational approaches, was born.

In order to develop this workshop, it was necessary first to evaluate the current education systems and biases of programs used to educate therapists and teachers themselves. While for many years therapy and education were described as both art and science, a belief system emerged among professionals that supported only the scientific side of clinical and educational programs. The "art" side of therapy has become only superficially acknowledged, with little attention to the importance of assisting clinicians in developing skill and accuracy in this component of an effective treatment program. Students and practicing therapists and teachers are educated and trained in a fact-based approach, with the assumption that through our teaching and clinical practice we must be able to explain everything we do rationally, and as much as possible must be explicable by scientific theory and research. Hence throughout their own education therapists and educators have had extensive experience with the rational model for gathering and interpreting information—a scientific model that reaches its conclusions in a linear fashion after considering each piece of data. For example, the therapist or educator observes each aspect of the client's disabilities and then moves in a step-by-step fashion toward the conclusion. Only information that "makes sense" and can be verified objectively is included.

The second requirement was to find the existing models of thinking that would validate an intuitive-rational model. The terms "intuition" and "clinical intuition" might be substituted for the old term "art therapy." An intuitive approach to assessment and treatment is based on "hunches" and on spatial timing components of the session.

We may define intuition as "knowing something without knowing how we know it." When using our intuition, we open all of our physical and non-physical senses in obtaining a global impression of the child and family. We may ask specific questions of our intuitive self and wait for the answers as we continue our work. This intuitive data may be refined and specific points checked out by more specific questions and observations. The clinician responds strongly to subtle non-verbal messages and an intuitive knowledge or hunch that either promotes further investigation or leads directly to a conclusion. Changes in space and time occur so easily and appropriately that therapy exhibits an aliveness and a flow from one event to the next.

We discover that information does not initially have to make sense to be considered in the conclusion, for making sense out of something usually implies that it has been subjected to a rational analysis. Much of the information utilized within the intuitive approach cannot be validated objectively at the time it is perceived to be accurate.

The intuitive approach leads to quantum leaps in understanding. It is an essential component of creativity. It allows us to become more sensitive to our own needs and to those of the children and adults working with us. It improves the effectiveness of our clinical problem-solving.

Recent brain research provides some of the support for the intuitive-rational model. Investigation of right-left-hemisphere specialization or processing preferences has revealed multiple ways of dealing with information for learning. The styles represented by the right hemisphere (intuitive, spontaneous, holistic, visual, artistic, spatial, non-verbal, symbolic, diffuse, playful) are equal to the processing styles of the left hemisphere (analytical, linear, sequential, verbal, concrete, rational, goal-oriented). Through the integration of the two hemispheres and the integration of cortical processing with subcortical, we have full access to our total capability. There is now greater acknowledgement of the role of subcortical areas of the brain in learning and problem solving, particularly in the reticular formation which centrally regulates sensory input and in the limbic system which is the seat of emotions and memory storage. Research also indicates the possibility that initiation of action is subcortical rather than cortical, as has always been presumed. Some researchers also feel that intuition and creativity may have major links with the limbic system.

When we are skilled and efficient in bringing into play all styles and ways of understanding a situation or concept—globally/intuitively, linearly/rationally, emotionally/cognitively—we can say, metaphorically at least, that we are using our whole brain. Hence we might consider the whole-brain concept, particularly right-left-hemisphere styles, as a metaphor for education and therapy. If we honor only the scientific and rational, ignoring the value of the global and intuitive, we are using only half our capacity as human beings. We honor the processing styles of the left hemisphere and ignore those of the right. If we use only the cognitive and ignore the emotional, we are honoring the processing contributions of the cortex and ignoring those of the subcortex. We are most complete as learners, and as human beings, when we bring our total capacity into play.

As we work with children, adults, and families with special needs, it is valuable to integrate rational and intuitive styles of thinking and problem-solving. In so doing, we bring together, honor, and teach both the science and the art of therapy. To do this, we must have skill and confidence in both ways of processing information. Hitherto, professional experience, with its rational-linear mode of teaching, has implied that intuitive thinking is inappropriate in the therapy and educational processes. Yet most professionals and parents engage in intuitive thinking as they deal with the daily issues that confront them. Most bring aspects of intuition into the therapy or classrooms. However, because of the bias which we have been taught, few have developed their intuitive skills to as great a degree as their rational skills. Because of its known effect on creating a more equal balance of energy in the two hemispheres of the brain, and the effect of emotional balance through the subcortical limbic system, Hemi-Sync creates the natural environment for developing this blending of intuition and rational processing skills.

With these considerations in mind, a workshop was designed to enhance the development of clinical intuition. This three-day program utilizes elements of the Monroe Outreach workshop, combined with practical application exercises and discussions, to create a model for blending and integrating rational and intuitive information. Participants in the first four workshops have included professionals in special education, speech-language pathology, occupational therapy, physical therapy, therapeutic riding, and music education. Several parents of children with disability have also taken part.

The goals of each workshop are to assist the participants in the following ways:

To discover and trust their own particular perceptive and intuitive skills;

To create a receptive mode for learning and gathering information;

To become more sensitive to their own inner needs and those of their clients;

To improve the effectiveness of their clinical problem-solving; and

To rapidly gain access to intuitive states of consciousness which support creative thinking.

The design includes a careful blending of rational and experiential components. These can be summarized under five headings.

A. Understanding of Intuition.

Participants are led to develop a greater rational understanding of different types of intuition and intuitive messages, on the physical, emotional, mental, and spiritual levels. Various situations in which intuitive thinking occurs with greater ease and accuracy are discussed.

B. Understanding of Hemi-Sync and Ways in which It Supports Intuition.

This includes discussion of the construction of the signals and a summary of the basic and applied research. Participants have a first experience of Hemi-Sync in a group setting, followed by discussion of its relationship to enhancement of intuition.

C. Tools for Accessing and Using Intuition.

Participants listen to eight Hemi-Sync exercises and discuss ways of using the preparatory tools. They experience the different states of Focus 10 and 12, including the exercises dealing with emotional cleansing and problem solving. Interwoven with the tape experiences are a series of practical discussions and group exercises to practice and affirm the use of intuition with another person and to create applications in therapy and educational settings.

D. Application of Hemi-Sync with Children.

Videotapes and discussion on the use of Hemi-Sync in enhancing sensory integration, developing focus of attention, increasing learning skills, and developing self-esteem in adolescents are presented, with information on the advantages of the process and guidelines for use with others. Participants are able to see that the children and adults with whom they work could be responding to Hemi-Sync in the same way they do. This raises the possibility that we can help these children develop a stronger intuitive knowledge of their own needs and learning process. When both therapist-educator and child are operating out of a strong intuitive space, the joint knowledge of direction for the program will be enhanced.

E. Continued Application Practice After the Workshop.

Two workshop manuals are provided. One contains information and references on intuition and space to record experiences during the workshop. It includes further ideas for playful practice in intuitive thinking and a format for more formally evaluating the correctness of intuition for those desiring a more structured approach. The other contains a series of papers on Hemi-Sync and the learning environment and a set of evaluation forms that can be use with children and their families when Hemi-Sync is employed. Each participant takes home the tape *Moment of Revelation* and the group sets a date to listen to this together at home. This provides a link back to the shared experience in the familiar home setting.

Follow-up questionnaires reveal that participants find greater willingness to use and trust their intuition in their personal and professional lives, and many report greater accuracy in meeting the needs of children and parents. Almost all were continuing to use the tapes for themselves, and over three-quarters of those who responded were using Hemi-Sync in their work with others. These "others" included infants, children, adolescents, and adults of all ages and can be divided into four groups:

1. Persons with a disability, including diagnoses of cerebral palsy, learning disabilities, hyperactivity, mental retardation, autism, sensory integrative dysfunction, receptive and expressive language disorders, emotional disturbance, and anxiety disorders;

2. Normal pre-school children in an integrated classroom;

3. Parents of children with special needs; and

4. Other teachers and therapists.

The settings for use included individual therapy, school classroom, home-based infant program, hospital, and rehabilitation center.

The tapes were used in several different ways:

1. As background for therapy or classroom activities;

2. As background music in the home for meals or preparation for the day's activities;

3. While writing reports and therapy notes;

4. For specific relaxation and concentration activities;

5. At bedtime to assist sleep;

6. For guided imagery sessions for brain-damaged adults;

7. To reduce negative behaviors in children.

The results observed included the following:

1. Increased willingness to accept sensory stimulation;

2. Decreased emotional outburst and increased ability to shift tasks;

3. Greater language fluency;

4. Greater relaxation of teachers and staff working with the children;

5. Children more emotionally relaxed and open to suggestions and changes in routine;

6. Easier bedtime routine, with children falling asleep more easily and parents also getting more sleep;

7. Nurses in the hospital more relaxed and calmer with the children;

8. A reduction in self-stimulated behaviors;

9. Increased ability to stay focused and pay attention;

10. Improved grading and control of movement in physical therapy;

11. Easier and more rapid completion of reports and therapy notes.

Experience with the workshops to date show that intuitive skills can be taught successfully and relatively rapidly, and that this learning may be enhanced when Hemi-Sync is used as a tool. The workshop model, blending experiential intuitive experiences with logical discussion and analysis of the intuitive process and tool application, created a model for blending the rational and intuitive. It is one thing to increase your intuition and another to learn to use it and blend it in an environment in which rationality is expected.

Some participants had already established a meditative or spiritual practice that used similar but different tools to reach states of awareness facilitated by Focus 10 and 12. They preferred to continue with their familiar route rather than use tools learned during the workshop. Some were unprepared for the power of the Hemi-Sync process in enhancing their abilities to explore within themselves and this created a barrier that needed to be overcome. Most felt they were somewhat intuitive at the beginning of the workshop but because of their professional training they had learned to hide this ability or to notice it only in their personal lives. The validation of their intuition, enabling them to trust and introduce it into their professional activities, was perhaps the most notable aspect of the program. One participant put as follows:

> The workshop affirmed the value of my intuitive style and helped me to value and trust my intuition more. I have also become better able to retrace my intuitive processing to be able to explain it in rational terms (e.g., I can look back and analyze what information I was picking up on in the situation). I no longer feel the need to apologize for using intuition as part of an effective decision-making process.

Two responses to the question "What in your opinion was the most valuable aspect of the workshop?" complete this account.

> The validation of myself as an individual with incredible untapped inner resources that at some level I felt were there but generally neglected in order to attend to the logical and acceptable. It made me feel much more valuable as a part of all that is: one part of our universe—having energy that connects me to all and provides a way for me to contribute.

> I now acknowledge parts of my being which I bring to life experiences, and especially to my work, that have never been clearly named or encouraged before. I feel more relaxed and

trusting in my abilities, in the grace and wonder of encountering another human being in my work and the recognition of a process under way, and in an exploration of ways to make communication easier.

What Right Have We? Ethical Considerations and Other Reflections

Gregory D. Carroll, Ph.D.

In 1985 Professor Carroll, Professor of Music at the University of North Carolina at Greensboro, conducted research on the effectiveness of hemispheric synchronization as a learning tool. The following is adapted from an Appendix to his report.

From the information that has been amassed through professional applications, the positive impact of Hemi-Sync technology for the individual and for society in general appears to be considerable. Within education, anecdotal reports and a handful of pilot studies suggest practical and promising benefits. However, in spite of these preliminary results, difficulty and resistance arise when attempts are made to assess scientifically its potential in the classroom.

The institution of public education in the U.S.A. is an immobile structure—based upon a nineteenth-century cultural model—resistant to significantly different and new ideas. When attempts are made to introduce this technology in the classroom, one of the first questions often asked concerns the "right" of the researcher (or anyone else, for that matter) to induce changes in the brain-wave patterns of another person. While I am not an authority in the areas of ethics or philosophy, I would like to share my thoughts on this matter.

What "right" does a person have to alter the brain-wave activity of another? This question arises when discussion of possible classroom use is undertaken with educators, school administrators, and those unfamiliar with the Hemi-Sync technology. It presupposes that each of us is in some way in control of such patterns, when in fact we usually are not. Our brain-wave activity, for the most part, is controlled by outside stimulation. We respond to external stimuli in the world around us, most of the time on a non-conscious level. If, for example, a driver cuts sharply in front of our car during rush-hour traffic, we do not respond by thinking about the changes produced in our brain's electrical patterns! We do, however, experience a sense of sudden shock, followed by anger and nervous tension. We are not in control of how our brains operate on the biochemical/electrical level.

More specifically, in the classroom the teacher and the environment are major factors affecting the student's brain-mind state. An energetic and motivating teacher, by his or her very presence and effective teaching style, produces changes in the electrical patterns of the students' brains that are conducive to successful learning. The teacher is able to elicit focused attention and concentration because he or she assists the students to generate the appropriate brain-wave patterns. In contrast, a hot classroom in the afternoon coupled with an uninspiring and monotonous instructor will induce brain patterns in the students which lull them to sleep.

What right does a teacher have to provide a visually pleasant and stimulating classroom decor? What right does a teacher have to provide a motivating atmosphere for learning? What right does a teacher have to provide students with these basics for successful learning experiences if it affects their brain waves? The point is, we do it all the time! Teachers who don't do these things lose their jobs.

What right do we have to provide a sonic environment that may assist in the focusing of student attention? Perhaps we are asking the wrong question. What right do we have not to explore a technology that may be beneficial to all students' learning? In these times, when students are herded through a system based upon fixed "seat time" with variable learning, and when "students' rights" are such an important issue, is it not a student's right to ask for or be granted a technology that will assist him or her in their educational endeavors? The only difference between what we are doing now and what we can do (in researching the effectiveness of Hemi-Sync in the classroom) is that the current standard methods of teaching, for better or worse, are sanctioned as time-honored techniques.

There is a pervading fear in our society of things that are new and different, or of things we don't understand. We are creatures of habit who find security in the status quo. We are habituated to habit. Now, to the ordinary person, Hemi-Sync may smack of a new technology with the potential for going berserk. It might evoke images of George Orwell's *1984* scenario as a means of "controlling" another person's mind or thoughts. Such misguided thinking has been a stumbling block in gaining approval of the technique for classroom use. But no one's thoughts can be "controlled" by Hemi-Sync. More than two decades of research and investigation show that these signals can be objectively and subjectively rejected by the listener. For this reason there was variance in the learning curves of students in the experimental group of my controlled study. The binaural audio stimulation of Hemi-Sync is not a panacea; rather it appears to be a useful tool—a part of a holistic classroom learning package—to enhance the learning environment.

With any technology there seems to come the possibility of abuse. We are aware of subliminal advertising in the cinema and the manipulation of society through advertising and political "sound bites." Billions of dollars are spent in order to control the purchasing patterns of large segments of our society. But there is nothing subliminal in Hemi-Sync technology, and no way has yet come to light in which it might be used to affect the mind of the listener without his cooperation and consent.

Hemi-Sync is not a "brainwashing" device. There is no text behind the signals. Within an academic setting, Hemi-Sync signals mixed with soft music or pink noise provide only an ambience—an environment—for potentially enhanced learning, sensitivity, and awareness. Successful learning is predicated on successful and effective teaching styles. If brainwashing is going on in the classroom it is due to the person in front of the class, not the technology creating the environment. And let us not forget that the teacher is also performing in the same acoustic habitat.

As scientists begin to examine more closely the relationship between music and the brain and the neurophysiological responses to audio stimulation, perhaps they will be less reluctant to consider research into the Hemi-Sync effect. As for researchers in education, we need to be free to do these studies now. We need to be free to ascertain the strengths and limitations of this technology. It may be more effective for certain learning contents and strategies than for others. We need to have controlled studies performed with the results framed in the language and protocol understandable to social and educational scientists. And if it proves to be only half as beneficial as the pioneering research data and anecdotal reports seem to indicate, we will have a responsibility to incorporate, in some way, Hemi-Sync in the classroom.

Learning To Fly

Cheryl O. Williams

Cheryl Williams, who was the first woman to coach an Olympic swimming team, signed on in the fall of 1991 to obtain her FAA Private Pilot License. She describes here how she incorporated the H-PLUS process into her training.

As I had only twenty weeks to devote to pilot training, I needed to get down to work immediately. Never having enjoyed mathematics, I knew that one of my greatest challenges would be mastering the calculations necessary to pass both the written and the practical exams. Having long accepted the premises that "we are what we think" and "thoughts are things," I decided to use the H-PLUS *Buy the Numbers* exercise. At first this had no effect, until I recalled that I normally began this process by using the "Plus Relax" and "Plus Focus" commands and then adding what I specifically needed. From then on I found that I could hold my attention on the math exercises and cope with almost all of the calculations on the course.

While I was studying for the examination, I played the *Concentration* tape continuously on my personal stereo tape player, as well as activating several H-PLUS functions linked together. I used the appropriate commands to deal with my limiting beliefs that I had poor mathematical ability. On the morning of the written examination, I reviewed all of the material, using the *Concentration* tape, took a nap (with *Catnapper*), and then drove to the center to take the test in the afternoon. Before the session began I listened to Metamusic *Inner Journey* and activated seven Function Commands in succession. I was quite calm and free of anxiety as I began the test. I worked for two hours on the computer test module. My results showed that although I did not score 100 percent, most of my calculations were correct and I had passed altogether with flying colors.

The practical part of the test, I realized, would be rather more complicated. I decided to continue using H-PLUS; each time I flew with my instructor and he presented me with a new skill to learn or challenge to overcome, I chained together seven commands to help me relax and learn.

The weather was perfect for my first solo flight. I told my instructor I was ready to go and he left me to taxi the Cessna 152 to the end of the runway. Before I ran through my checklist, I activated six commands to help me relax, think clearly, and synchronize mind and body. Then I opened the throttle and moved off. As the plane lifted off the ground, I knew for a moment the suspension of time and place. I felt free and excited, realizing that I had mastered the aircraft, the wind, and the laws of flight. I flew over the airfield and across Lake Erie; then I joined the air traffic pattern of the airfield to prepare for landing. Taxiing toward my instructor, I saw him smiling broadly. He told me to repeat the experience, completing one more circuit around the airfield. When I finally landed and taxied in, my instructor congratulated me—I beamed with pride!

Lessons continued, the hours of flying time were carefully logged, and new skills were learned. Each time I would use H-PLUS functions to encode the new learning. This helped me to become more relaxed and confident. My instructor asked me how I was able to assimilate new information so quickly, and I gave him a brief overview of the Hemi-Sync process. Now I was enjoying cross-country solos, landing at new airfields and moving on to different destinations.

One day while I was performing maneuvers with my instructor, he put the plane into a spin and told me to recover to level flight. I did this with confidence. Then he put a hood over my eyes so that my view was obstructed and the only way to control the plane was by observing the instruments and gauges. I managed this easily, and as we returned to the hangar after the lesson my instructor told me that he knew I was ready for the final test and he had already scheduled my "check ride" with the examiner later that day.

With some hours to get my thoughts together, I drove to the shore of Lake Erie and walked on the beach, listening to *Inner Journey* on my tape player and enjoying the experience. Returning to the airfield, I activated my six "flying" commands and began my pre-flight check. Confidently and easily I moved from one skill to the next as the FAA examiner tested me in the air. Then I heard him say, "Well, you've done a fine job. Let's go back to the hangar." I landed the plane—yet I knew my consciousness was still flying up there above the clouds—and walked with a spring in my step as the examiner handed me my license and wished me well.

Applications: Spirit

Chapter 5

Healing the Injured Spirit

Many psychologists and psychotherapists are now using the hemispheric synchronization technology as an adjunct to their work with clients. With scarcely an exception, all the practitioners and their clients who have utilized it feel that it is helpful, sometimes dramatically so, and the more they use it the more they discover about its potential. Other therapists employ the process as an element in their own courses and workshops in areas such as teaching stress reduction and controlling eating disorders, as an aid to pregnancy massage, in pre-birth instruction, and as an accompaniment to past-life therapy.

In this chapter, we look at the work of five practitioners, each of whom has researched the tapes and the sound signals and has determined how best to use them in accordance with his or her own approach. The chapter concludes with a discussion by Dr. Mohammad Sadigh on the reasons the hemispheric synchronization process is proving of such benefit in psychotherapy.

Effective Help With the Psycho-Spiritual Quest

Joseph Gallenberger, Ph.D.

Dr. Gallenberger is a clinical psychologist practicing in Hendersonville, North Carolina. He is also a trainer for The Monroe Institute.

In recent years, clients and their insurance companies have been asking for treatment to be completed as quickly as possible. This presents a challenge as therapy, in my view, needs to be a learning experience for the client, not simply an exercise in temporary symptom relief. I have sought to meet this challenge by using, where appropriate, hemispheric synchronization tapes, with the expectation that these would increase the clients' self-understanding while shortening the courses of treatment. To my surprise, this technology has also proved effective in dramatically increasing clients' spiritual progress. This article gives a few examples of how this method has worked in the past three years. Names and circumstances have been modified to guard confidentiality.

Ann had suffered from extreme claustrophobia for the past thirty years. When she was a child, her father had held her head under water in the toilet as a punishment. Her mother was anxious, critical, and controlling. She had also been trapped in two fires; once at school when she had taken refuge in a locker and was not rescued until the locker was filled with smoke, and the second time when she was trapped in a skyscraper. Now she found herself unable to enter confined spaces, such as an elevator, or to fly in an airplane.

Ann was referred for hypnosis. It was essential that she have a Magnetic Resonance Imaging (MRI) test to check for a brain tumor. This involves remaining motionless inside a very cramped tube for hours as the machine takes pictures of the brain. Many people who normally have no difficulty with small spaces have intense anxiety reactions in the MRI, and the use of anesthetics is not desirable as the MRI interferes with monitoring the patient's vital signs. The MRI team reported that no one even moderately claustrophobic had ever completed the test, and Ann had already tried and failed despite calming medication.

We met for twelve one-hour sessions in three weeks. To begin with, Ann dreaded the thought of hours motionless and alone in the MRI, although she was motivated for change. We started with the H-PLUS exercises *Relax, Let Go* and *Off-Loading*, and two tapes incorporating visualization. She practiced with them diligently. After a week, we began to use the H-PLUS format to enter a light, relaxed hypnotic state during alternating sessions. Here we explored in more detail the origins of her fear of being trapped, and used imagery to rehearse successful completion of the MRI test. Images of being surrounded by protective white light and of mentally expanding the space around her seemed particularly useful.

Throughout her adult life, Ann had not dared to dance or laugh because such acts were too spontaneous and could, she feared, bring ridicule. The interpretation that she had actually trapped herself by being so careful to please everyone seemed to make sense to her and helped shift the emphasis away from the dimensions of physical space, allowing her to see claustrophobia as a symbol of her internal state—trapped and fearing loss of control. She became determined to conquer this self-imposed restriction.

With this re-formulation, the battle became a spiritual one. Ann's concept of God, modeled after her father, was of an unforgiving and possibly sadistic being. Her concept of herself was of someone deeply unworthy, deserving of sorrow, and having little control. She feared that the MRI, if completed, would reveal an inoperable tumor and would confirm that God judged her unworthy of life. Her Creator was going to "finish her off" with a brain tumor. Then she would face final judgment and condemnation. The current crisis clarified and intensified life-long spiritual themes for her. There was no escape.

Three weeks after meeting Ann, I accompanied her to the MRI at a hospital forty miles from her home. The test was delayed for two hours, and the roads outside were icing over, yet she remained only moderately anxious. When the test began, she used the H-PLUS commands to "relax" and "let go" and she relaxed visibly, feeling confident that she would make it. At her request, I read to her from *The Tao of Pooh* to link her with the outside world and to give her something positive to focus on. The Taoist concept of harmonizing with life-energy had been introduced to her earlier.

Ann was successful this time, without needing medication. She reported feeling two minutes of ill-ease, then entering into a deeply relaxed state and eventually going to sleep. She, the staff, and I were all amazed at her accomplishment. Shortly afterwards she managed to conquer her fear of elevators, feeling that now she could master any fear. She also began to work on her fear of God and of her own nature. Her liberation from the latter fears was even more exhilarating to her than the objective victories she experienced.

I have no doubt that the tapes helped to establish a deep therapy alliance more quickly than would otherwise have happened. They gave Ann rapid control and allowed her to reach and "off-load" repressed material speedily and safely. This was more remarkable given that she had a lifelong history of understandable distrust, pessimism, self-harshness, and low self-confidence. Her triumph over the MRI left her eager to explore other aspects of her life and to make many positive changes. Her struggle and victory highlight the mystery of physical and spiritual interaction. Later Ann used the Emergency Series to help deal with the brain surgery that it was discovered she needed. These tapes seemed to reduce the usual disorientation and discouragement of such surgery.

The Monroe technology and other ways of quickly integrating the body, mind, and spirit can be used within the psychotherapeutic process to facilitate completion of the work. Without rapid and effective tools, therapy may become bogged down. Resistance, discouragement, and lack of power to implement change tax client and therapist alike. If working through these challenges takes a long time, the client may become too depleted in energy and finances to continue and to integrate the spiritual element. Metaphysical exploration may seem a luxury that is not affordable. In reality, the spiritual dimension may be the means of making worthwhile the whole experience of life-unhappiness that resulted in therapy. Spiritual issues themselves may fuel much unhappiness; yet this is usually veiled in our current cultural climate.

The pattern of trauma and recovery is a sad one unless there is meaning beyond typical therapeutic reductionism: "He hurt me because his father hurt him—all I can do is reduce the hurt inside me and stop it from being passed on." And the New Age point of view that "my own higher self arranged or permitted it, to work through Karma" can also be victimizing.

A rich spirituality, which celebrates the connectedness, love, and mystery found in ourselves and the universe and which affirms that the voyage through the labyrinth that humans experience is a sacred voyage, can be the true prize of the therapeutic quest. Alleviation of pain becomes only an important guidepost, not the end point of therapy work.

Since working with Ann, I have used the Monroe materials clinically with excellent success in various situations. Children with learning disabilities and/or attention deficits have responded very well to *Super Sleep*. Most attention-disordered children sleep very restlessly and have to re-assemble all their bedding each morning. With this tape playing all night, the bedding is intact in the morning, and both parents and teachers report improved concentration and less irritability during the day. These children often find difficulty in listening to relaxation tapes because they are so restless, but they tolerate *Super Sleep*, which does not require the same degree of stillness and concentration as it entrains them to a normal sleep-cycle pattern.

I have worked with several asthmatic children and adults with much success, using the H-PLUS *Lungs: Repair & Maintenance* exercise. One client in particular illustrated some of the complexities. This was a woman who had difficulty climbing a short set of stairs and was using an inhaler about six times a day. She seemed to be choking on rage generated by involvement with a series of abusive men. Within three weeks of using this tape, re-formulating her issues and taking assertive action to obtain more nurturance for herself, she was swimming a third of a mile a day and was seldom using her inhaler. This gain remained consistent over a one-year period. Again we see spiritual issues: letting go of anger, the trusting and opening to receiving, in this case breath and love. When therapy closes with an emphasis on clients' spiritual growth issues, it seems that they are more likely to report even years later that growth has continued and they are living lives of deeper joy.

In contrast, I have used H-PLUS *Strong-Quick* with two weightlifters who were refusing to dispense with the use of steroids for fear of losing their edge. Most weightlifters work themselves into an aggressive state for peak performance. I suggested using *Strong-Quick* with the image of pulling powerful energy up from the earth and then becoming a conduit for that energy. Both weightlifters reported being able to lift more weight than their best performance using steroids. They also observed an increase of smoothness and felt they had less potential for injury. This is a clear example of a physical/mental situation that provides opportunity for spiritual growth. The person is challenged to become aware of his connection with energy through an initial struggle to dominate his world.

Certain H-PLUS tapes have proved very helpful in marital situations, including spouse abuse, sexual dysfunction, and communication problems. *Empathizing, Speak Up, Let Go,* and *Off-Loading* are those I generally use. Abusers report rapid anger control. Clinical alliance deepens quickly with these men who are usually hard to treat owing to shame, skepticism, and their lack of self-control. Helping these men become aware of the meaningfulness of their issues helps restore their sense of humanity. Many men suffering from impotency and/or premature ejaculation have become more assertive and less performance-pressured within three weeks of using these tapes as an adjunct to therapy. What has greatly impressed me is that these strategies are effective even when the spouse refuses to join the client for therapy, which often happens in abuse and sexual dysfunction situations. When I do see couples together, I suggest they use these exercises before dealing with each other in session. The improvement in communication is striking. There is more listening, less accusation and defensiveness, and a far greater willingness to solve problems.

I have found that the most useful tapes for psychotherapy are *Let Go* and *Off-Loading.* They reduce fear and resistance and allow more rapid softening of long-held negative patterns of thought. The tapes have worked well with the majority of clients in my practice, including some usually difficult groups such as the resistant teenager, the passive/dependent, the obsessive, the psychosomatic, and the sociopathic. Most resistance has come from Vietnam combat veterans, paranoid personalities, and the "yes but" psychosomatizers. Of course, any client's reluctance is wholly respected; however, quickly clarifying a client's resistance can be very useful therapeutically.

Severe depression may be the most wretched malady man can suffer. Those who are depressed may feel isolated from all love and may blame themselves totally for their own feelings of helplessness and hopelessness, while the spiritual person may feel that in-dwelling Light has vanished. While an individual is clinically depressed I avoid the H-PLUS tapes because they require active participation and concentration. Instead I provide them with one or two Metamusic tapes. Many depressed clients report that this flowing, quiet music, with relaxing, balancing sound signals embedded in it, provides them with strong temporary relief and consolation and gradually helps in lifting their depression.

In addition to the H-PLUS series, the Gateway Experience tapes have also proved very helpful, especially with clients seeking to access their total self or to achieve age regression. Pete, for example, was a young man of tremendous potential who had been badly burned as a toddler and had the impression this was caused by his own clumsiness. His parents divorced shortly afterwards, and the family was reluctant to discuss his accident. He needed to re-experience the burn to find out what had actually happened, and this we were able to do by using the tapes to achieve a deeply meditative state. I then suggested that he was completely free of time, that he was at the center of a huge wheel, and that he could go to any time-period he wished by simply traveling down a spoke of the wheel. He immediately went to the burn episode. He re-experienced the episode in clear and close detail and with tolerable distress. He discovered that the accident was no fault of his and, more importantly, that when he had been released from hospital his relatives, fearing to injure his tender skin, had pulled away from him when he ran to embrace them. At that young age he could not handle this "rejection." Re-experiencing this allowed him to make rapid progress on many rejection-related issues in his adult life. Understanding the episode helped release him from low self-confidence and enabled him to begin to fulfil his potential.

A final example points out the powerful entrainment effects of the Hemi-Sync process. Once exposed to enhanced awareness during tape-listening, the "altered state" is often easily replicated without the use of a tape. This potentiates the utilization of enhanced awareness during daily life.

Beth was a bright, hard-driving middle manager, severely hampered at her job by budgetary and political pressures. She had been in therapy for two months and was using the Gateway tapes at home. She came to a session very angry and distressed, wanting to be able to enter a meditative state and get answers to questions but too upset to do so. Having talked through some of her problems, I suggested that she take a breath and move herself into the state of high awareness she had been experiencing while listening to the tapes at home—and seek high-quality answers to her concerns. I then asked her five relevant questions to which she obtained immediate answers which we both felt were profound and on target. This gave her a sense of a quantum leap in control and expanded her definition of self. She saw how she could employ the same technique at work during the difficult parts of her business day. Together we contemplated how it would be if major political and business leaders used such access to higher self when faced with important decisions.

As a therapist, I have found it to be deeply satisfying to have a new tool which seems so safe and effective. It has helped me to be a better therapist, and my confidence and enjoyment in my work have increased. Neither clients nor therapists enjoy wallowing in the negativity of the discovery phase of therapy, and often feel rather lost as to how to implement changes rapidly and effectively once the desired changes are targeted. The Monroe tapes can help to shorten the unpleasant and uncertain phases of therapy, leaving more time and resources for growth, for discovery and celebration of one's worth, and for increasing one's contribution to the world. Hemispheric synchronization is a twenty-first-century tool, allowing a smooth integration of technology with compassion and clinical skill. Because no belief system other than "we are more than our physical bodies" is required, it can be incorporated into most schools of therapy, whether ego-analytic, existential, humanistic, behavioral, or transpersonal, enhancing rather than straining the modality. It answers the need for rapid results while illuminating the humanity of the client and the therapist.

We start with a spiritual yearning, but find ourselves struggling with darkness. In my opinion, organized religion provides a candle. But it is often hard to see past the candle's light—the religious dogma. Traditional meditation techniques are like a lantern. They extend awareness but have their own distracting light and still only dimly illuminate the ineffable, because without years of practice they tend to produce results erratically.

Hemi-Sync is analogous to a halogen flashlight. One can see with greater reliability and precision and without distraction from a dogmatic light-source. Yet Hemi-Sync is only an elegant tool. It makes no sense to stare directly at the tool for any length of time. And it doesn't instruct you where to point the light it provides. It invites you to access your own in-dwelling wisdom about this important step. That's where the magic of the spirit comes back in!

Fertile Inner States
Laura Batchelor, M.A.

Laura Batchelor is an educational therapist practicing in St. Louis, Missouri, specializing in Jungian theory, creative/vocational expression, spiritual development, and transitions. Here she describes her work with new clients.

I often find that new clients

a. Live in an agitated state; they have forgotten or are not consciously aware of a relaxed mental state. Typical methods of evoking relaxation are sexual activity, alcohol, drugs, food, and sleep.

b. View their lives through a body consciousness, an emotional consciousness, or many of the other forms that cultural, rational consciousness takes.

c. Lack conscious experience of their own dreams, visions, active imagination, or creative visualization.

d. Feel that the state of "mind awake/body asleep" has no value. Most often when it occurs for them it is viewed as a lack of sleep.

e. Perceive the use of intuition or objective consciousness as too assertive, controlling, or illegal or as a weird state of mind not to be trusted.

f. Have a very low tolerance for the higher vibratory levels that conscious attention can induce.

Generally, I will introduce a client to the hemispheric synchronization process when there is a call for reduction of stress and anxiety. After an initial and often lengthy discussion of relaxation methods, I ask whether the client has used any kind of sound techniques and if there is any interest in trying one for stress reduction as well as to aid the present work of balancing right and left brain functioning.

Most choose to use the tape. First I introduce them to The Monroe Institute's work and describe Frequency Following Response and hemispheric synchronization using the explanations from the Institute's brochure. Then I provide the tape—initially I use *The Way of Hemi-Sync* and the "Are Thoughts Really Things?" pamphlet, which cites the application of a topographic display EEG computer system to investigate the relationship between brain waves and states of consciousness. Finally we discuss equipment, preparations for listening and scheduling, and the broader application of learning about other energy systems. The client takes the tape and literature home and is responsible for deciding how often and when to use the tape.

Out of the first twenty-five clients introduced to this method, twenty-four immediately decided to use the tape and the other one requested it later. Three returned the tape, one saying that "in a home of six children there was no undisturbed time to use it" (he now uses Metamusic for the whole household to hear), and the other two said their ears were too sensitive to the sound. Two others, while they feel that this is a very good application for them, had trouble finding time to listen to the tape.

Ten clients use the tape frequently. Eight have started the Gateway Experience home course, while others have gone on to the H-PLUS function exercises and the Metamusic series.

I find that, for clients, use of Hemi-Sync

a. Reduces stress immediately, allowing the mind to focus on work to be done in the session.

b. Often provides a new experience.

c. Begins to orient the mind to giving pleasure to the entire organism.

d. Provokes thinking of new means of relaxation.

e. Gives the mind a reference point for re-creating the whole-brain state.

f. Gives the mind permission to talk about inner, primary learning system behavior.

g. Evens out emotional highs and lows. As one client states, it brings him to a centeredness in which he can be more objective about himself. Without this, there seems to be a tendency to focus on negatives.

h. Begins the development of an effective attitude for problem solving and creative adventure.

Frequently I notice an interesting and surprising reaction to the introductory discussion about Hemi-Sync. Clients will often respond with what seems to be a newly found excitement, hope, or anticipation. In following conversations they will describe these initial responses as the point at which they consciously began to feel relief from the psychoemotional pain they were experiencing and the lessening of superfluous mental chatter.

I find *The Way of Hemi-Sync* tape a most valuable tool for establishing a fertile inner state—a state which evokes a necessary step toward understanding how self-criticism and conscious self-reflection impact the psyche. This understanding, achieved bit by bit, leads toward a broader comprehension of self and fosters the ability to control attitudes and thoughts deliberately. Thus, the client is able to become aware of, and thereby utilize, the fields of energy within and outside of the psyche.

Before I introduced Hemi-Sync, most of my work was on the personal, five-sensory level of consciousness. Since its introduction, all except my newest clients work on the intuitive level, in the multisensory area. With the lessening of the repression of the intuitive and universal levels of consciousness, those engaged in the individuation process are now able, with their newly discovered multisensory personalities, to explore progressively farther reaches of their physical and non-physical beings. In recent months many clients have told me that dreams, never thought possible a year ago, are now coming true—thanks to much hard work and this new therapeutic tool.

I find that, in Carl Jung's words, "Many of my cases are not suffering from any clinically definable neurosis, but more from the senselessness and aimlessness of their lives." Jung suggested that this state of being seems to be a form of the universal neurosis of our time—a time in which fundamental values are dangerously wavering and a spiritual and psychic disorientation has taken hold. In view of this, I submit that the "way of individuation" as postulated by Jung and the "way of Hemi-Sync" as offered by Monroe are two excellent ideas, each informing the other of the possibilities of what is, and what can be, manifest in this world.

"Something Has Happened"

James M. Thomas, Ph.D.

James M. Thomas is a clinical psychologist working in Ponca City, an oil town in Oklahoma, where his patients include many oil men, engineers and scientists who, he finds, often have difficulty getting in touch with their feelings. When they come to him, he says, most of his clients want more options, some sort of experience (they want to know "something has happened"), and something that they themselves can do. For many, "if you haven't helped them on their very first visit, they won't be back." Hemi-Sync helps greatly to meet these needs, as may be seen from his report.

Before using a Monroe tape, I brief my clients on the content and outline the possible results, with suggestions of the benefits they are likely to receive. A generally useful suggestion is that listening to the tape will give clients the opportunity to learn something about themselves, which is especially appealing to teenagers. I prefer that clients listen to the tapes in my office, operating the equipment themselves and thus involving them to some extent in their own healing process. Most of those who come to me are over fifty years of age and the majority of them report some degree of physical pain. I often begin with *Introduction to Focus 10* (Discovery 2), which includes a thorough and detailed relaxation exercise. This usually helps to decrease the sensation of pain, leading to fuller relaxation.

As a result of my experience, I have found that Hemi-Sync has three main benefits. It increases the all-important rapport with a client; it enriches a client's dream content and improves recall; and it activates memory (especially repressed memories). I have discovered that the most useful tape overall is *Introduction to Focus 10*, although it has not helped with cases of drug or alcohol abuse or with schizophrenic clients. However, *Concentration* could be effective with schizophrenics and borderline personalities, as well as being useful for "pulling people together." *Catnapper* helps with

PMS and general anxiety, and also with those suffering from extended jet lag. I also use exercises from the H-PLUS series; others that are useful include *Color Breathing* (Threshold 4) and *Mission Night* (Exploring 4), which helps with sleeping problems.

I am a consultant for the Department of Human Services and the local American Legion Children's Home, whose director of social services is Charles Danley. Having obtained permission from the administration to use Hemi-Sync in the Home, which accommodates about fifty children of veterans, ranging in age from ten to seventeen, who have been removed from their homes and whose basic nature is generalized as "aggressive," Mr. Danley constructed partitioned listening booths and provided cassette players and tapes. The tapes included *Introduction to Focus 10*, *Catnapper*, *Concentration*, *Cable Car*, and *Crystal Fantasy* (a non-Monroe tape played through the synthesizer). During the first trial period, a rating of the children's behavior was made on a Behavioral Rating Scale, ranging from 0 to 10—with 0 indicating the worst behavior and 10 the best. Thirty-nine days after the period began, the average rating for the group increased from 2.87 to 8.27.

A further study was undertaken with the eight "worst" children, all classified as "seriously emotionally disturbed." They were asked to read the Gateway Affirmation and to listen to *Introduction to Focus 10* three times a week for eight weeks. The incident reports of this group fell to less than half of the pre-study reports and remained significantly lower in the succeeding weeks. Walkmans and tapes are kept available for use by children when they feel especially tense or liable to "blow up."

Future plans for the Home now include the installation of built-in speakers and headphone outlets in new dormitories and a proposal to include a protocol for the use of Hemi-Sync in every child's Service Plan (the contract between the state, the child, the Home, and me), together with the issue of a handbook for parents explaining the process.

A Research Project

Sylvia Perera, M.A.

Sylvia Perera is a Jungian psychoanalyst in private practice in New York City and in Sherman, Connecticut. She teaches at the C.G. Jung Institute of New York and is the author of several books. She used Hemi-Sync in sessions with five patients for a month-long "research" period to try to estimate what effects it might have. Here is her report.

I prepared the clients differently for the use of a mechanical adjunct to the usual therapy and I noted individual results. In all cases, however, there was a marked change in my feeling relaxed, alert and centered, which must have had an impact on the therapeutic field. There was also increased client ability to perceive and to verbalize what I am now calling "derivative messages of balance." These messages were particularly noteworthy in two borderline clients. The tendency to split perceptions and emotions into mutually exclusive either/or states is part of the borderline diagnostic picture. But the same effect occurred with a manic-depressive female client and a male with severe compulsive and intellectualizing defenses.

One borderline woman with a history of self-mutilation and psychotic ideation came into the session in panic, feeling paranoid that "a man had been watching" her on the train. I was playing *Surf* with appropriate signals at a level just below traffic noise so it was not really audible. She gave no indication that she was aware of it. I remained silent except for a brief question to elicit the objective facts about her experience on the train. She began to relax after about twenty minutes of whimpering like a fearful infant, alternating with hypervigilant arousal and urges to hurt herself again. She then said, "I can begin to relax into my body. I can begin to feel safe. . .Oh, I can see something double. Feeling safe and being watched and hated can be together! That's weird. That never happened before." In a later session with the same signals, she talked about "feeling real in a space we share—not alone in terror. You are there—here too. I can be with you together."

A manic-depressive hysteroid woman in the first session when I used Hemi-Sync remembered a dream of "standing between two men, so I am not afraid." She then spoke more coherently than usual, with less manic anxiety. Later in the same session she provided a derivative message of balance quite explicitly by talking about "balances [she could feel] between light and dark parts of [her] body, above and below." At another session she reported she could get "an overview [of her sense] of shame."

With the intellectualizing male client I tried a signal to induce deep relaxation to attempt to outflank his normal conceptualizing persona. We both nearly went to sleep. During six sessions of this state, we were mutually able to experience and acknowledge the power of nearly autistic defenses under his previous glib, left-brain talk. Exploring these deeper defenses led into memories of the abuses that had walled off his vivid emotional life in early childhood. About three months later, I tried different signals and he responded immediately by talking about "balancing conceptual and emotional sides" of himself.

To a severely phobic client I urged the use of the *Deep Ten Relaxation* tape. After using it a few times with what he reported as positive results, he lost it. This provided analytic material to begin to analyze the grip—and secondary gains—of the phobic responses. Another client refused to use the tape at home, feeling I was shoving her off with a surrogate caretaker, as her mother had done by leaving her with maids. But she has responded well to Hemi-Sync in sessions with me. Hemi-Sync seems to help her to process her dependency cravings more realistically.

These are anecdotal data. It is impossible for me to do anything more hardline experimental with living clients in an intentionally therapeutic field—even though therapy by its very nature is somewhat experimental and improvisational. For example, I cannot tell how much of the effects were due to the Hemi-Sync sounds on the clients or, as I indicated, how much they helped me to stay centered and objective as a research observer and thus affected the mutual field. In either case, I do think there was a benefit. And with the particular borderline woman referred to, I attribute her slow but radical shift to that month of sustained use of the technology. I chose to use it after three years of work with her. Why that moment felt "right" and why and when I choose to use Hemi-Sync with which clients is something about which I am still musing. It may be that there is a need to explore fully the nonbalanced states until I have an intuition that a synthesizing stage is appropriate.

Since that month of research, I have been using Hemi-Sync quite intuitively. It is very hard to know what exactly is going on in such a complex, multidimensional field as psychotherapy, especially as the observer here is part of the field.

Two Case Studies
Dwight Eaton, Th.D.,Ph.D.

Dr. Dwight Eaton is a clinical psychologist practicing in Honolulu.

"The terrors that spring from our elaborate civilization are proving to be far more threatening than those that primitive people attributed to demons," maintained Carl Jung. "That is why finding the inner meaning of life is more important to the individual than anything else. And why the process of individuation must be given top priority." The impetus for this is found in another of his statements: "Part of the unconscious consists of a multitude of temporarily obscured thoughts, impressions and images that—in spite of being lost—continue to influence our conscious minds."

I found that it was possible for a patient listening to the phased sound signals through headphones to be able to move into these "temporarily obscured thoughts, impressions and images" and to arrive at the primal cause of experienced events in half an hour or so, a process which might take months or even years using conventional methods.

Case Study #1

Subject: Female, early 30s; Caucasian; employed as a stripper in numerous local night clubs.

The subject first presented in response to a suggestion from a prior client in the same profession. Her stated initial reason dealt with the physical abuse she was then experiencing from her current paramour. Extensive history-taking revealed repetitive occurrences of physical and psychological abusive treatment from former spouses and live-in boyfriends.

The subject had been earning a comfortable living for at least twelve years as a nude performer in various clubs in the United States

171

and in Asia, at one point engaging in live sex acts with one of her former husbands. To begin with, she expressed great admiration for her chosen profession and lifestyle. Heavy use of drugs and alcohol were also a part of her daily regimen. She was attractive and bright and appeared well-adjusted. Her deep-seated contempt for women generally became evident in numerous subtle ways. Her own quite poorly developed and negative self-esteem was most apparent. The first exposure to Hemi-Sync produced a reported sense of great calmness and relaxation, plus a "miraculous" recovery from the effects of a previous night of "binging."

The following week, again exposed to Hemi-Sync, she experienced a most vivid "dream," the recall of which was taped. With no suggestion from me, during the week between the second and third visits she chose to write down the details of this encounter, a summary of which now follows.

She recalled being a fifty-year-old man, named Amok [a most significant psychological disclosure, at no time revealed to the subject by me, the definition of which is ". . .a psychic disturbance characterized by depression followed by a manic urge to murder"], living in a very cold and desolate area probably somewhere in Asia in the 1700s.

Amok had a wife and two daughters, a sled, twelve dogs, and necessary survival paraphernalia. While traveling with his dog team to take some frozen meat to relatives, among whom was an eight-year-old girl, he encountered a violent snowstorm. Abandoning his team and sled, he took shelter in a cave whose entrance became blocked with blowing snow. As he had previously done with his own two daughters, he abandoned his twelve dogs. Amok said, in effect, "I did little to show my appreciation. I mainly separated myself from women, which I did by focusing on myself."

Amok continued, "I froze to death in that cave and I had murdered my twelve faithful dogs. I left the cave [immediately after his death] to view the scene. My dogs were dead, frozen in the snow drifts. I remember my heart felt like a stone. It couldn't feel a thing for the dead dogs—my ego would not let it. My wife was scared and worried for me but I cared little or nothing about her well-being."

The subject commented, "My past life experience as Amok has been a very humbling experience for me. I am far less quick to judge others, for example, my father" [who also abused her]. Others in the field of psychiatry will appreciate her unconscious tendency to select male companions who will abuse her; her lifelong fear of dogs; her contempt for females; prejudices and selfishness; being actually quite lazy and begrudging her work choice; dissatisfaction with her own body; offended by her own body odor; and having abandoned her real-life daughters because "they failed to give me the ego-boost I desired." She continued, "I was not grateful for much in my life. . .my attitude reflected this. I wouldn't allow myself to feel much joy. . .my ungrateful attitude was my prison [cave?]. . .I judged the physical and ignored the spiritual. . .I measured my worth by material things."

At the time of this writing, the subject has voluntarily given up her accustomed means of livelihood and has secured employment in a large local drafting firm.

Case History #2

Subject: Male, age 35; Caucasian; professional bartender; seven-year resident of Hawaii.

Subject presented quite recently with a complex of sex-related dysfunctions, most anecdotal, one clinical. The clinical history is the excision of a single testis some five years previous due to a suspected carcinomal incursion. No recurrence, extension, or experienced inhibition to date.

From his earliest recollection, the subject entertained profound doubts as to whether he was "straight" or "gay." On the many occasions in his adult life when he attempted intercourse with a woman each attempt followed an identical pattern: initial rigidity followed by immediate flaccidity resulting in non-penetration. Hence failure followed by bouts of embarrassment, shame, disgust, and self-loathing.

Attempting to compensate for these failures, he early commenced the solicitation of selected white males in a limited manner, wishing to stroke and be stroked and to experience being the recipient of fellatio. He consistently refrained from reciprocal performance or involvement in penetration. He declared a repeated profound disgust and self-loathing in these actions. His usual method of relief consisted of regular masturbation. This suggested the absence of physical impedance as to competence in erection, maintaining rigidity, and ejaculation.

The subject exhibited numerous kinesthetic symptoms: chain smoking; constant changes in attitude while standing or sitting; clipped, quick speech; nervous and consistent knee-bouncing while sitting; finger tapping; and nervous laughter, but only when appropriate.

Testing failed to suggest any evidence of psychoses, fugues or phobias. It appeared to me that he was experiencing a complexity of allied dysfunctions possibly stemming from a single traumatic event buried in the unconscious, which exhibited solely at the emotional level when triggered by related mechanisms.

Using standard deep-level hypnosis techniques employing focusing, suggestions, relaxation modes, and so on, I tested the subject for creative visualization propensity. This was successful in that it helped to calm him down and diminish his kinesthetic symptoms.

In the next session, I introduced him to Hemi-Sync with exposure to an Alpha signal. During the review following the session, he disclosed that he had made a date with a female patron and mentioned, with some trepidation, that a sexual liaison had been intimated. I suggested that, should the occasion arise, he share with his companion a brief outline of his previous failures in an attempt to elicit her understanding and cooperation. This he did, reporting that, for the first time, he had experienced a completed sex act with a woman. Subsequently he found that he occasionally reverted to his old pattern of failure, inducing the customary negative emotions.

During a later session, the subject was exposed to a Hemi-Sync "deep relaxation" signal, having been previously instructed to concentrate on the sounds and to repeat rhythmically the thought, "What event caused my condition?" After thirty minutes he reported, emphatically and excitedly, that he had had a most vivid dream of an event which took place when he was twelve years of age involving his elder brother of fourteen. He had not recalled this particular event since its occurrence, but had just experienced it in its entirety.

Early one morning he was alone in the house with his brother, whom he greatly admired. His brother invited him into his room and showed him his erect penis, asking him to caress it. He did so, and experienced immediate disgust, shame, and embarrassment, and instant and total disintegration of all the values he had previously held for his elder brother. The event was never again mentioned by either and was forgotten by the subject until this exposure to Hemi-Sync. Conventional hypnosis had failed to assist him in re-creating this critical event. Hemi-Sync is proving, beyond doubt, a valuable procedure for demonstrating Freud's important dictum: "To relieve 'it,' 'it' must be relived."

A subject does not need to suffer for months, or in many cases years, the rigors of conventional therapies in order to arrive at the primal causes of experienced events. I feel that this subject, with continued work using Hemi-Sync, will soon be capable of experiencing a "normal" sex life. The conclusions that may be drawn from this single event are perhaps too complex and myriad to be included in a report of this nature, but those in the practice of psychotherapy will recognize them.

Insight-Oriented Psychotherapy

Mohammad R. Sadigh, Ph.D.

Dr. Mohammad Sadigh is Director of Psychology and Psychophysiological services at the Gateway Institute, a center for pain and stress management in Bethlehem, Pennsylvania. He is in charge of the center's neuropsychological laboratory. His primary research activity is in the area of computer-assisted brainmapping.

While it is becoming more and more clear that the Hemi-Sync process is of benefit in psychotherapy, we need to address the question as to why this should be. How does hemispheric synchronization contribute to the psychotherapeutic process? In this article, I will attempt to offer a theoretical explanation, supported by some preliminary research findings.

Insight-oriented psychotherapy is based on the premise that psychological, emotional, and behavioral problems and difficulties originate from unresolved unconscious conflicts left behind from our childhood years. These unconscious conflicts continue to affect us—our relationships, our careers, and ultimately our perception of reality—unless they are acknowledged and dealt with. The goal of psychotherapy is to make these unconscious conflicts conscious so that we may gain control over them. Theoretically speaking, once this is accomplished we are no longer victims of these unconscious forces, and our reality is no longer tainted and distorted by these determinants of behavior which normally operate outside our conscious awareness. Unfortunately, however, accomplishing this task fully is extremely difficult and in most cases almost impossible. The patient and the psychotherapist often have to grapple and struggle with a variety of conscious and unconscious defensive barriers and practical limitations, which make the process long and emotionally (as well as financially) exhausting. Yet psychotherapy cannot be effective without understanding and dealing with such unconscious defenses and what erected them in the first place.

A simple example illustrates how unconscious conflicts and defenses are formed and how they may affect a person's life. Imagine a scared child who is given a highly conflicting message by her mother as she enters her parents' room looking for security and comfort. On entering the room the child hears the verbal message (left hemisphere) "I really want you to stay here with us," while at the same time she also "hears" the facial expression which says (right hemisphere), "I wish you would go to your room so that we could sleep in peace without you." The left hemisphere hears an inviting, pleasing message, while the right hemisphere "hears" rejection, and experiences sadness and emotional pain. These wholly conflicting messages may seriously impair the child's ability to respond to her mother. Her only way out is if and when one of the messages is blocked or pushed outside the realm of conscious awareness. As Freud (1916) said, "Defense is always against affect." That is, if the material perceived by the right hemisphere (which is affective in nature) is defended against, the child is likely to go on and behave normally for the time being.

Although the child may appear to have resolved the emotional and perceptual conflict of the moment, it is very possible that the seeds of doubt, mistrust, and confusion have already been planted in her mind. As she continues to deny, block, and repress her inconsistent perceptions, she experiences greater turmoil and tension within. In other words, the nonverbal material in the right hemisphere, even though submerged in the subconscious, will continue to have a life of its own and will, at one point, manifest itself in the form of physical and/or psychological symptoms.

To put it differently, lack of validation and communication between the two hemispheres may result in the construction of defenses which, in time, could alienate the child from herself. These unconscious barriers are apt to isolate and stop her from recognizing and acknowledging her resources, abilities, potentials, and propensities that could easily save her from emotional and psychological torment and make problem-solving a manageable task. Hence, we come to witness the birth of "mental and physical disorders" and psychosomatic symptoms and conditions.

Early in his work, Freud (1913) discovered that, by allowing them to free-associate, his patients were able to uncover some of the unconscious material that was interfering with their normal functioning. Symptoms, both physical and psychological, began to disappear slowly as the unconscious became more conscious. Today, free association continues to be a potent tool for conducting insight-oriented psychotherapy. It appears that, during the free-association process, important information and material tend to seep through the defensive barriers spontaneously. This results in recognition and realization of determinants of behaviors, conflicts, and traumas often locked in the dungeons of the unconscious. But again, because of the complexities of defense mechanisms, this process is often time-consuming and extremely exhausting. Theoretically, the process of psychotherapy can be accelerated should the two hemispheres begin to communicate more freely with each other and transcend the defensive barriers.

In seeking to discover how we may facilitate this communication, I began to study the effects of the Hemi-Sync process on cortical activity. In study after study, I was able to demonstrate objectively that Hemi-Sync does indeed do what it is claimed to do: synchronize the two hemispheres of the brain. What are the implications of this interhemispheric synchronization? Once I recovered from the euphoria of observing synchronized brain states after exposure to Hemi-Sync signals, I began to explore what was happening cognitively, as well as affectively, to each subject.

The results of my pilot studies have been promising. In the first two studies, while psychotherapy patients were exposed to Hemi-Sync signals they were asked to free-associate—that is, to talk about whatever came into their minds. In both cases, from an objective standpoint (monitoring cortical activity), two observations were made. Initially there was a tendency toward intrahemispheric synchronization followed by brief episodes of total bilateral synchrony. During these moments of whole-brain synchrony subjects often had an "aha" or "clarity" experience. Based on these observations, I have come to believe that one of the many states that Hemi-Sync facilitates is that of hemispheric communication (Hemi-Com) or, perhaps, as a psychotherapist would put it, "an integration of content and affect." This, to a large extent, is what psychotherapy is all about, and it is remarkable to observe that Hemi-Sync may indeed facilitate and expedite such a process.

A number of ground-breaking papers stating that meditation played an important role in psychotherapy (e.g., Smith 1976) appeared in psychotherapy journals in the late seventies. Their authors, however, failed to propose a convincing explanation for why or how meditation contributed to the psychotherapeutic process. At last, it appears that we may have an answer. In our neurophysiological laboratory we have already demonstrated that experienced meditators tend to synchronize their brains. More recently we are beginning to see that moments of bilateral synchrony coincide with moments of "clarity." Hence it may be that the reason meditation is such an important tool in facilitating psychotherapy is that it promotes whole-brain synchrony; it opens a channel of communication between the two hemispheres which may allow certain "unconscious" defenses to be transcended. If we can systematically and consistently demonstrate this process of hemispheric communication in more elaborate and well-controlled studies—that is, hemispheric synchrony followed by clarification of affect and thoughts—I believe we will be making a giant leap toward better understanding of how the human mind operates and how to facilitate its healing.

References

Freud, S. 1916. *The Unconscious*. Standard Edition 14:159-204.

Freud, S. 1913. *On Beginning the Treatment*. Standard Edition 12:121-144.

Smith, J. 1976. "Psychotherapeutic Effects of Transcendental Meditation with Controls of Expectation of Relief and Daily Sitting." *Journal of Consulting and Clinical Psychology*. 44:630-637.

Chapter 6

Transcendence: The Spirit on High

As the hand held before the eye conceals the greatest moun-
tain, so the little earthly life hides from the glance the enormous
lights and mysteries of which the world is full, and he who can
draw it away from before his eyes, as one draws away a hand,
beholds the great shining of the inner worlds.
Rabbi Nachman (1772-1810)

Many listeners of the Monroe tapes report that they have had experiences of a transcendent nature, similar to the "peak experiences" that Abraham Maslow describes in *Towards a Psychology of Being*. Such experiences may occur to anyone at any time, with or without some external stimulus: in meditation, during a religious service, while walking in the countryside, or at any moment in the daily round. Psychologist Dr. Darlene Miller says that many of those with whom she has talked at The Monroe Institute have had one or more such experiences without using Hemi-Sync, but adds that it seems Hemi-Sync "somehow enhances and increases the frequency of these occurrences, that with its use they are more controlled rather than spontaneous happenings." These are not "out-of-body" experiences, which characteristically involve traveling and a different mode of perception, but experiences which might be described as mystical or transcendental.

There are, says Dr. Miller, certain common factors that frequently occur in reports of these experiences by Hemi-Sync listeners. They are (1) being bathed in white light, (2) being surrounded by a dark expanse filled with millions of stars, (3) feeling a "loving presence" around or in them, (4) having an awareness of greater energies of which they are an integral part, (5) feeling deep peacefulness and joy, (6) gaining an understanding of the "oneness" of all things, and (7) the perception of the dissolving of all boundaries and limitations.

In the Institute laboratory there is an isolation booth where the individual lies on a water bed filled with a mixture of salt and water approximating to the consistency of the Dead Sea. The booth is so constructed that the interior is totally sealed from outside influence and the temperature is a constant 91.3 degrees F. After a few minutes, the subject is unaware of where skin ends and the world beyond begins. The sense of physical identity is lost, and the subject becomes a point source of consciousness. Whatever is experienced comes from inside the head. If signals are being relayed, the experience may be induced or deepened by the Hemi-Sync tone patterns. The subject is in communication via headphones and a microphone with a monitor outside the booth, and body temperature, galvanic skin response, and potential skin voltage are recorded on computer throughout the session. These readings give some indication of the degree of relaxation and the psychological involvement of the subject with what is happening and can be correlated with the experience being undergone, which is being reported and recorded on tape. For research purposes, the subject may also be connected to a twenty-channel Neuromapper, a sophisticated EEG device linked to a computer which produces topographic maps of the electrical activity in the cerebral cortices.

Sessions in the booth may be used for personal growth and development, for obtaining technical information, or in what is described as the "explorer mode," where the subject acts as an open and willing receiver of knowledge, ideas, information, or experiences that might not be gained in any other way. Recordings of some of these sessions are available from the Institute. While the content of some sessions may be practical and matter-of-fact, others may give rise to a type of "peak experience" as described above.

These "transcendent" experiences, no matter where or how they are received, are unforgettable and sometimes extremely powerful. What follows is a small selection to give some idea of their nature and variety.

Three Experiences

Laura was attending a Gateway program and found after three days that she needed to become more active in the process if she was to benefit more fully. This is how she describes what happened:

My decision to become active helped me to cooperate with the powerful audio signals in the first Focus 12 tape. It was so powerful for my physical system that I automatically switched to rapid breathing to keep up with the force that I was feeling. It was both thrust and pull. My body felt like a rocket under jet propulsion while at the same time my head was being pulled with magnetic force, up and up and up. Everything stilled, and I sensed myself lying on my back, arched over the curvature of the earth, looking up into the infinitesimal blackness. Light flashes much like electrical short circuit sparks emitted on both sides of my peripheral vision. As I looked into the blackness which had a depth that didn't end, I sensed that I was experiencing what infinity is like. . .

On the last day of the program there was an exercise with no sound signals, only Bob Monroe's voice guiding the participants through the process. Laura continues:

I arrived at Focus 12 without difficulty. Since I was not feeling creative enough to have a "purpose" for this free-for-all, I asked, "Do you have a message for me?"

A "voice" said, "Love your neighbor, dear Laura."

My Christian upbringing made this message "old hat." I knew my understanding must be limited, so I asked, "Can you be more specific?" The top of my head began to pulsate and expand upward and outward until it felt like a universe. As the pulsation continued, I experienced a new oneness with this "universe" and a new appreciation of "Christ Consciousness."

Bob's voice broke in to suggest we go on to Focus 15, the state where time to the experiencer does not exist. The pulsing of my head stopped, and it took surprisingly little effort to arrive at that familiar place. Without my asking, the "voice" said, "I have loved thee from all eternity." My chest began to pulsate and the love within became intense. . .loving what I felt was my Creator and being loved in mutuality, not just at the moment but from the Beginning. I had a new understanding of the "I am." I felt a tear trickle down my cheek and fall into my ear. This was an unconditional love that I had never known before.

Bob's voice called for us to return to Focus 10. My thumping chest subsided. A reluctant but easy descent followed, but the message was not finished. In one insightful vision, I saw many key incidents in my lifetime, all quite diverse and unrelated, flash together under a common theme. Whenever I felt a loss, or even subconsciously sensed impending loss, with someone wanting what I didn't want to give, I had patterned my behavior to pull back and say in effect, "No, it's mine." (My physical integrity, my possessions, my time, etc.) Until now I had not been able to identify this fear. It was hidden under "justifiable" responses. Now with this flash of insight in seeing my fear of "loss" in operation, I was able to release it with pleasure. Simultaneous with this new understanding came the return of the pulsation, head and chest moving at the same time. The trinity of love completed, I knew I had to break this pattern of withholding what I have and what I am.

Just before the session, our trainer, Melissa, had admired a very favorite sweater of mine and I jokingly asked her if she wanted it. Now I knew that I had to give it to her, a symbol of my new-found freedom. There was a momentary thought of, "Well, I'll wear it today and give it to her tomorrow." The next thought was more compelling: "Awaken with the Beta signal, take it off, go downstairs, and give it to her without delay." She didn't want to accept it, of course; I could only insist, "You must—it's energy conversion."

What has persisted over time is a feeling of acceptance of others wherever they are in their evolution or attainment, or lack of it, which has eliminated a lot of judgmental thoughts.

* * * * *

Sara was at home, lying on her bed in a darkened room listening to the Open Exercise *tape, when she began to get a sense of vibration and movement. She describes what followed.*

I began to feel a great sense of energy and also a sense of no presence of my body. It was such an unusual experience that I opened my eyes and could see the darkened room well enough, but still I had no sense of body. It was as though my eyes looking out were the edge of my self.

What I sensed was a vast sea of atomic matter, or consciousness, or energy matter, with which I was wholly intertwined—that there was quite literally no separation between my self and the universe. It was as if it were all a sort of soup of consciousness in which "I" was merely a point of focus, or a point of view, a sort of a twitch in this infinite web of energy. Also the sense of "point" was as the concept is described in mathematics, in which a point has no dimension, no space, only location. There was understanding intuitively that this is the circumstance of all consciousness or even any physical object; that it is merely a point, an idea or pattern about which atoms have been drawn.

The exquisite thing about this experience was that it was not an abstract idea—it was a very real experience, one that is accessible to me as part of the human collection of "real" experiences.

Although I have had another intensively mystical experience previously without the tapes, and although I am quite interested in these sorts of things, I had not gone into that tape seeking such an experience; it just happened. Experiences such as these seem so magnificent and exquisite and affect one so profoundly, yet are so ineffable.

* * * * *

David describes a session in the laboratory isolation booth, which produced a physiological response that so far cannot be explained. He was lying on the water bed when he felt that he was being "washed with waves of unconditional love." The waves, which felt like "warm honey," began at his head and washed throughout his entire body. It was to him a physical as well as a psychological sensation, as if he was immersed in vibrating waves of energy.

As the experience continued, he became aware of unaccustomed sounds in his headphones—muttered comments and giggling. When he emerged from the booth, the monitor and the technician who had been observing the read-outs of his physiological state on the computer screen asked him what had been going on. He described the experience as well as he could and asked them in turn what had been amusing them. They told him that at the exact time when he reported the "waves of unconditional love" the physiological read-out of his skin potential voltage showed that he was creating absolutely square waves—like the crenallations on a fortified tower—something that was theoretically impossible for a human being to do.

Since then, four more people have been found who under certain circumstances of enhanced awareness have produced similar square waves. More research is needed before any tentative conclusions can be drawn, but David's "square waves" are interesting as a hitherto unrecorded physiological response to a transcendent type of experience that may one day find its place in the scientific literature.

The Out-of-Body Experience

In recent years, the kind of experience now usually described as "out-of-body" has become generally recognized as unquestionably valid and frequently of great value to the experiencer. In *Far Journeys*, Robert Monroe describes the out-of-body experience (OBE) as "a condition where you find yourself outside of your physical body, fully conscious and able to perceive and act as if you were functioning physically, with several exceptions. You can move through space (and time?)...You can observe, participate in events, make willful decisions based upon what you perceive and do. You can move through physical matter...without effort or effect."

It would appear that OBEs are much more common than was once thought; indeed, when the subject is raised it seems that almost everyone can describe the condition from their own recollection. Listening to a Hemi-Sync tape may sometimes stimulate such an experience. However, if achieving an OBE is the sole motive for tape use, unless you are an adept at moving into the OBE state you are very likely to be disappointed.

While many OBEs take the experiencer on journeys that in "everyday reality" he could in no way accomplish within the time frame available, some—like the one that follows—may move him no further than the next room.

The Living Body Map

Keith D. Clark, M.A., D.C.H.

I am thirty-five years of age, a clinical hypnotherapist and professor of Interpersonal and Organizational Communication.

I am also classified as a quadriplegic. Nine years ago, I fractured my 3/4/5 cervical vertebrae in a body-surfing accident. This resulted in an initial diagnosis of what is termed "a complete injury," which means I had no sensation or level of control below the level of the injury.

Perhaps an easier way to relate this is to imagine having your arms extended out at your sides, parallel to the ground, and then drawing a straight line from the index finger of one hand to the index finger of the other. Everything below that line, including the fingers, is basically asleep, or outside of conscious control or feeling. This diagnosis is readily accepted as irreversible.

So much for my personal background. What I am now endeavoring to do is to use words to describe an experience which is far more powerful than any language. I ask the reader to keep in mind that, while it is widely accepted that our choice of words becomes the experience, this experience was well beyond the scope of language.

One weekend in the fall of 1991, I had the opportunity to participate in an Outreach workshop. I was in the company of several friends, teachers, and other like-minded people. There were twelve of us in all.

We started the tapes on Friday evening, continuing through Saturday and Sunday morning. We all enjoyed a weekend full of experiences, sharing, and fellowship. I felt a bit removed from the group when we listened to the tapes but only because of the physical distance. The others were all gathered in the main room, lying on floor mats, while I opted to use an adjacent room with a bed in it. Throughout the weekend, the energy in the building was fantastic.

On Saturday evening, I was lying on the bed listening to the *Living Body Map* tape through headphones. I began to have an ever-increas-

187

ing sense of power, and then lightness. As I was becoming aware of this, I also sensed a freedom—a freedom and ease of movement. It was indeed freedom from the long-felt constraints of the paralysis that my body had been subjected to for the past nine years.

Gently and smoothly, with great intention, I sat upright. And, it what seemed so effortless a way, I rose to my feet. With a brief hesitation, I carefully took my first step. Well, perhaps it wasn't a step but more of a shuffle. But at any rate I was standing erect. Not only was I standing, but I had movement!

As I began, slowly and cautiously, to move toward the door, I became more confident in my ability to move effortlessly—as effortlessly as anyone does who has not experienced a mobility impairment, in the way we all take movement for granted until we are deprived of it.

I was fully experiencing all the sensations of my body. I felt the texture of the carpet beneath my feet—the carpet which I had seen but never felt before. I was aware of the subtle feeling of the air across my arm as it swung forward when I took another step—this time lifting my foot.

I raised my arm, perhaps instinctively, opening my fingers to brace myself against the wall. Instantly I was aware of the cool temperature of the wall, and of its solidity and smoothness of texture. My sensory system had become awakened. I was being bombarded with sensations. My mind was racing to welcome all of the input connecting these seemingly new experiences with past experiences which had long lain dormant, waiting to be called upon once again. Present also was a mixture of emotions. I was elated but also cautious, and I even felt a slight air of disbelief.

I continued toward the doorway that led to my friends in the other room. I relished with delight each slow and deliberate step and movement. I was amazed how perfectly my body was once again responding to the requests I made of it.

Nevertheless, the ten or so steps that it took to reach the door seemed to take as many minutes. I was constantly concerned that something might give out or that I might fall. I thought that I would hate to fall and create a racket that would disturb the others.

My concerns were short-lived, however, as I finally reached the doorway. The excitement of moving from room to room caused me to forget them. A feeling of comfort and confidence came over me, not unlike the comfort one experiences when turning on a light switch on entering a pitch-dark room.

I moved quietly and effortlessly about the room so as not to disturb anyone listening to the same *Living Body Map* tape which had freed me to begin this new journey on a familiar path.

It was then that I turned toward my long-time friend and mentor who was leading the group. As I looked down upon her face, I had a sense of how tall I was. My injury had reduced me from my one-time height of six feet, two inches down to four feet, six inches—but now I had moved back again. As I continued looking down, I noticed that she was becoming more distant. Suddenly I realized that I was floating—that I was being led or taken to another place. A place that is here and now, while being beyond here and now.

And there I met with what I have heard the Hawaiians, and perhaps the Native Americans, refer to as "your Council."

At this point I don't know that any words can describe what happened. I do not recall any visual aspect of the meeting. There was no clear physical presence, nor was there any auditory channel. There was, however, definite communication. I would call this an "imparting of knowledge," and I was aware of a presence which our very limiting language might possibly describe as "an unlimited source of love."

It was my sense that this experience was not unlike the planting of a seed, the germination, growth, and flowering of which would take place in time. And in time my own understanding of the information would become usable and complete.

As I sensed myself still "out there," I insisted that I did not want to return into the confines of a paralyzed body. I was invoking my greatest volition to repair the body I was destined to return to. I was in an almost desperate frenzy, trying to bring back with me whatever would allow me to repair the damage to the physical body that I had chosen and was identified as belonging to me. I remember saying over and over again, "I am not going back without full recovery; I am not going back into physical limitations. . ." Then a bit of what I would call "a sense of caring parental reassurance" came over me—and I was back in my body.

As I lay there with eyes still closed, the tape was ending. Finally it stopped. I thought once again how I wanted to get up—simply to open my eyes and swing my legs up and over to the right, place my feet firmly on the floor, sit upright, and then stand.

I recalled how vivid the recent experience was. I searched my memories for other experiences of going from a reclining position to standing. I consoled myself that it was time to open my eyes and fully return to the building with the others who I could now hear beginning to move about.

As I opened my eyes and began to focus on the room, my legs began to move. And with one graceful movement both my right and left legs simultaneously swung up and over the right side of the bed. My feet were both placed firmly on the floor. My hips were in alignment, and from almost any angle it would appear that I was ready to get out of bed.

Now it is true that I did not physically stand that day. However, my body did respond in the exact way in which I had asked it to. This was the first time since my accident nine years before that I had intentionally moved my legs to exactly where I wanted them.

A week later I repeated the *Living Body Map* tape. I again finished the tape, opened my eyes, and moved my legs over, placing my feet once again upon the floor.

It has been several months now, and I appear to be getting stronger and increasing both in sensation and control of my body. I am not yet walking, but don't forget my name and keep an eye out for further information!

Note. The Living Body Map *exercise is designed to enable the listener to balance and strengthen the body, physically, emotionally and mentally, as well as recharge and energize it. Using a visualized map of the body the listener creates the perspective and detachment useful in healing. The principles of color therapy are also used in this exercise.*

The Transcendent Experience

The archives of the Alister Hardy Research Centre, Oxford, England, contain several thousand accounts of religious or spiritual experiences collected over the last twenty years. Many of them are set, like Laura's, in a specifically Christian context. There seems no doubt that the individual's own cultural or religious background creates the framework for the experience; research into religious experience in India reveals, naturally enough, that Hindus refer to Krishna, Kali, or the healing deity Venketeshwara Bhairava, as well as to "The God Almighty." Many of the "Monroe experiences" might have come from the Alister Hardy records. Not all, however; some bear resemblances to the world of science or space fiction, others carry echoes of the writings of Madame Blavatsky, Alice Miller, or those who channel the thoughts and words of various disembodied entities.

It would seem that such experiences, whether described as transcendent, religious, spiritual, or mystical, are more common than was once thought. Many people, however, are reluctant to discuss them for fear they may be misunderstood, not taken seriously, or even laughed at. Several of those who corresponded with the Alister Hardy Centre reported how disappointed they were with the reaction from ministers and doctors from whom they sought help and advice in coming to terms with what they had experienced. In contrast, those whose experience coincided with the use of Monroe tapes have always found sympathetic, helpful, and encouraging responses from the trainers, staff, and their fellow participants.

What happens in the brain when a "transcendent experience" occurs? Some would say it doesn't matter; such experiences have been reported since the earliest known records (there are several of them in the Bible, for instance) and they have been accepted on their own merits without the need for scientific enquiry or validation. In these times, however, with the increased interest in the investigation of consciousness and with the development of such devices as neuromappers, enquiry is proceeding whether it "matters" or not.

One investigator, who has been researching into consciousness for some fifteen years, is Dr. Edgar Wilson, a neurologist and founder of the Colorado Association for Psychophysiologic Research. He is especially interested in the transcendent, or dissociative, state and has recently been considering the effects of the Hemi-Sync technology on such states. Dr. Wilson's article in this chapter is his own account of his research, adapted from an address he gave in 1991. (Explanations of the technical terms may be found at the end of the article.) A brief technical report on a recent study Dr. Wilson undertook with six subjects is included in chapter seven.

The Transits of Consciousness

Edgar S. Wilson, M.D.

This is a personal story—a story of discovery. However, before I describe my recent work, let me share with you the historical context in which we look at consciousness. We look at consciousness through the eyes of electronics, of perspicuity, imagination, wonder and delight, and all of those things that go to make up the neat mysteries that surround the lives we live, if we care to open our eyes to them. This is perhaps a journey into mystery, a journey into our own unfolding, greasing the transits of our knowing.

I started researching into consciousness in the late 1970s at the University of Colorado in Boulder with David Joffe, a computer wizard. We were doing galvanic skin response and EEG on left and right brain, when this idea was new and folk thought the right brain did intuitive stuff and the left cognitive and that was that. So we had only two channels—and that was all we could see, right and left brain. However, the reality that unfolds before you totally depends on the shape and size of the window you are looking through—so our first findings confirmed our suspicions about the world as we constructed it.

Using the computer, we could record and analyze blood pressure and pulse, skin potential, and brain waves. In this way we could take people through a stress-profiling procedure. After many experiments, I found that stress-profiling didn't work for finding extraordinary or transcendent states of consciousness. It only showed instinctual, habitual responses of survival.

Nevertheless, we did find that we could take our computer readings and convert them into alpha, theta, high alpha, and low alpha, and we tried desperately to tag those on to states of consciousness. But this became confusing and troublesome; people would not do what we thought they should be doing. So here we were stuck trying to define all these squiggles on our charts and making little sense of them. Then David moved up to an XT386 computer and a math co-processor and we began to look at things up to 60 Hz, then up to 128 Hz—and people were busy up there too! But they shouldn't be—it's not in the literature; something called gamma stops about 40 Hz, we were told, but we were seeing people doing things up to 128 Hz, although we didn't know what or why.

We began to look at people in normal, wakeful states and again we found that they were constantly changing. They're not in beta, alpha, theta—they were in all of them and more, and they were shifting constantly. How do you make sense out of this? The more complex the people were, and the more tasks you had them doing, and the less defenses they had, the more this shifting occurred. We are apparently capable of processing very many things at once. You're not thinking just one thing as you sit there. A part is monitoring your gut gurgling after breakfast, a part is monitoring what I'm talking about, a part is making judgments about it, and other parts are doing a host of other things all at once.

In fact, after all my years of looking at this stuff, I have yet to find that consciousness even exists in the head. We may just be sending messages, commands, to set up the resonances to get the muscles moving, the digestive juices going, but we really don't live in our brain.

We seem to create a fundamental illusion of time and space by concentrating very narrow-focused alpha activity in the back of the head. This process creates the illusion of certainty because it temporarily overwhelms the seeming chaos of multiple stimuli. This allows us to concentrate on learned signals and values.

I started to find out about five years ago that sound made a noticeable difference to brain-wave patterns. I could get people to change with sounds. We began to see people change states of consciousness, particularly when I used binaural beat frequencies, which I'd heard about—a certain Robert Monroe had done this since 1957 but there were no references. Then I started giving the individual feedback with sound of his own brain waves. Now we could get him to track more than what there was beyond alpha; he began to do things with his brain waves that he should not have been able to according to the scientific literature. For example, the temporal lobes would light up in theta when listening to soul-moving music.

Another thing I found at this time was that I, as the researcher, had a profound effect on the actual outcome of the experiment I was running. So I began to work on myself. I began working with holotropic breathwork and hyperventilating to intense music and found that I had feelings, something I'd forgotten for thirty years. When you practice medicine you grow callouses around your soul so that you can tolerate the pain of other people. Opening that up was no small issue. When I began to feel again, my own brain waves changed. Now I could light up my temporal lobes. I had greased a transit I'd forgotten I had.

The research process began to unfold. To change their states of consciousness, people had to be free to follow their feelings. They had to feel this was legitimate; otherwise, all I recorded was novelty response—more alpha. Now, as I stimulated them with sound that encouraged emotion and feeling, I began to find changes that would occur in the brain as a direct response to the stimulus I was putting in.

I have also found a change in the electromagnetic field around the individual being studied during changes in his states of consciousness. With a Hemholtz coil placed one foot above the head, I found a shift in the electromagnetic field during a change within the subject from a high-alpha focused state to a low-frequency feeling state. During this time, a progressive increase in frequency and power occurred in the coil's activity, precisely coinciding with the internal change of the subject. This is the first scientific indication of Monroe's idea that we can exist outside our bodies.

That process led to an understanding about the first nature of transcendent experience. Time/space is the first thing to go when one is moving into a transcendent or dissociate state. Dissociate states occur when you lose time/space. It seems to happen right in the middle of the head—the crown chakra if you like—that starts to go off at the point of opening oneself to what is, instead of what ought to be in the future or what should have been in the past. It's the moment of "Aha—I exist in this moment—now, and now keeps changing. I can't go back, I can't go forward, I can only exist in this moment." And suddenly something starts to happen as time/space is transcended.

Next I started studying healers, and found that they tended to drive people into this time/space warp when they were working on them, if there was great congruence between the healer and the healee. One day Rod Campbell, a seventy-seven-year-old from New Zealand, came into town. He's an old cowpoke who discovered twenty-five years ago he had something about his hands that could transmit healing energy to others. He could reduce you to tears; he was so sincere; he had nothing to prove and he wasn't trying to make money. He was too simple, and simple people bothered me because I couldn't explain what they were doing. Rod would hold his hands over someone, who would feel warmth, vibration, energy moving, particularly if we put Rod in a more natural environment, such as a cabin in the mountains. There, where it was warm inside and the belief systems were congruent, the tears would start and suddenly something would change. We had brain-wave measuring apparatus on both subjects, and we would switch back and forth between the two, and I had a magnetometer above Rod's head. He made beautiful spikes of ascending frequency and power as he went into his healing mode. I'd say, "Rod you can heal him now," and he would do it; I'd say, "Rod you can stop," and he would. He said it just came through him. When he was working on someone, the subject's frequency would change, and change back when he'd finished. Rod was emitting high frequency and enormous activity, and everything else was shut down. Something was happening here, in very high frequencies, with no evidence in alpha, beta or theta. My rational mind is really boggled by all this—I keep trying to explain it away.

It seems that suddenly there's a shift from the center of the head out to the temporal areas as you go from the loss of time/space awareness to an awareness of deep empathy, those moments in our lives—only moments for most of us—when we lose the sense of separateness from each other and from our world. Those are the moments when we are able to strip away that last little vestige of fear, to know that we are part and parcel of the same stuff, transcendent stuff. And we see also that this is accompanied by low-frequency emissions, 1 to 6 Hz, in the center of the head. This seems to keep time/space at bay; it's almost as if we go to sleep to our past and our expectations. You get a higher frequency as you move into a transcendent state. There's a splitting, similar to what you would see in a paranoid personality who can't fit into our world, where he's not accepted for his splitting. How ironic it is that we, who are so frozen into our alpha state, trying to be appropriate, to learn everything there is to learn, are willing to come to The Monroe Institute to pay money to learn how to split!

In the healer experiments, this splitting occurred at a very profound level. At the time, I checked all Rod's physical functions (eye movement, respiration, heart rate), and none of them was active in affecting the brain waves. Rod was making deep, slow waves, drawing you down into a comfortable state—and then splitting you off where you could play. It was both weird and wonderful! That's where I was when I came here in November.

These phenomena, which would happen only in brief bursts, would occur with a really slow frequency to begin with and work their way up. The normal brain wave frequencies, delta, theta, alpha, beta, are hardly more than 2 microvolts power. Rod's frequencies—

18 to 32 Hz at 9.7 mv; 32 to 64 Hz at 29.9 mv; 64 to 128 Hz at 39 mv, were totally out of the range we'd ever looked at before. The temporal lobes alone are lit up—there's nothing holding the person down, no theta-delta—it's all in the temporal lobes in high frequency.

When I looked at the literature, I found that only Penfield had stimulated the right temporal lobe when doing brain surgery. Then the patient would talk about psychic phenomena, relate things that weren't there, such as out-of-body experiences, and so forth. In fact, the first reference to OBEs with temporal lobe stimulation was by Penfield. Later on, Baer thought that since temporal lobe seizures were often associated with transcendent experiences, OBEs, and other "psychotic type behaviors" that it was due to hyperconnectivity between the temporal lobe and the cortex, and he could demonstrate that the temporal lobe would light up in people with temporal lobe seizures.

Persinger showed that people answering a questionnaire that described temporal lobe seizures and disorders often had these esoteric experiences and OBEs. The questionnaire would just as beautifully define those who were having transcendent experiences and OBEs. We are in a world in which "transcendence" and "dissociation" describe two value systems about the same phenomenon. The distinction seems to be, however, that dissociation (as described by Persinger) is a state of low arousal which spreads from the temporal lobes throughout the brain, whereas transcendent experience is a state of high arousal within the temporal lobe area.

Interestingly, people who channel, who have psychical activity, but cannot remember the content of their channeling or their psychical experience, seem to light up the right temporal lobe only. Those that bring back the content of their experience seem to light up both left and right together.

When I arrived at The Monroe Institute I knew little about it. I was aware only that this was one of the few organizations which had established some kind of laboratory to study consciousness—that's what I'd been trying to do for several years—and it was one of the few labs actively doing anything in this area of research. Most of the university labs had shut down because nobody could define consciousness, or for some other petty excuse. When I arrived to look at the process, I found an enormous amount of data had been collected from the computer system, the brain-wave machine, etc. Nobody could make any sense out of this; so I sat down and said, "What is going on here—what could be going on?"

Now I want to share with you one of the most frenetic months

I've ever spent, looking at that process from as many ways as I could but failing to see any relationship between the signal they were putting in and what they were getting out. Listeners were obviously having some kind of transcendent experience and were describing very similar experiences, but I could see no evidence of it—only a normal EEG parameter. I decided to give up my expectancies and simply to watch to see what happened. This I did, and lo!—some fascinating things began to unfold.

As I observed, I found that putting in a signal was having some kind of an effect in the brain. When we matched up the frequency bands across the head, they would come in bursts until suddenly everything got together and the person would start having a state change. They would begin with really low frequencies, like low delta, followed by an escalation of frequency in a certain harmonic pattern. I tried to match this with harmonics like octaves, but it didn't match. However, the harmonic was a Fibonacci series, a series derived from Pythagoras, who made his reality a kind of progression of a series of numbers which for him represented something very spiritual. We see the Fibonacci series reproduced in plants' branching and in DNA and RNA. We see it as it progresses in the nervous system, the dendrites and neurons branching and unfolding from the deeper structures to the outer structures. The Fibonacci series is all over nature—why couldn't it be in the brain? Could this sacred geometry of Pythagoras apply to the way the nervous system processed sound?

So we experimented with the Fibonacci series and began to analyze these bursts, low frequencies going into higher and higher frequencies at the crown chakra, and we began to see they followed certain patterns. Waves swept out from low to high frequencies as the individual opened himself to a transcendent state. These waves were somewhat irregular and hard to pin down; however, what was apparent was that there was a reciprocal relationship going on here: that as the alpha frequencies decreased there was an increase in both the delta frequencies and these other very high frequencies. When alpha came back in, the higher frequencies were dampened. So alpha may act as an inhibition to the shifts into transcendent states.

We still don't know what generates brain waves—we know so little. We do know there's a kind of a pacemaker which makes the alpha; it's located very close to the fourth ventricle where the reticular activating system is, and that pacemaker seems to be associated with memory, which is very much state-dependent according to the frequency we're working in at the time we receive the information. So the memory is for externally imposed knowledge, educated knowledge. I find that people who are poorly educated but have great wisdom make very little alpha. Most people who have gone through graduate school make an enormous amount of alpha—they can't stop making alpha, it seems. And the more you fight your alpha the tighter it gets, the more rational the man becomes.

Alpha seems to be the timer by which we frame our time/space reality. When we let go of alpha we go into a more immediate awareness of what is in this moment, not what we expect it to be. So this splitting phenomenon is a shift away from this time consciousness into a space-opening consciousness. The split is maintained by holding a very low-frequency/high-amplitude activity in one part of the brain, and then shifting up into the temporal lobes. I found this true in healing and in psychic and channeling experiments. We have discovered a common pathway. Up to now there's been no stimulus that can be consistently called upon to explain the phenomenon. You have a phenomenon here that you can predictably and comfortably stimulate by using a binaural beat stimulus. What I'd been looking at before was generally a happenchance phenomenon that occurred or didn't, depending on the congruence of the belief system of those participating.

What else occurs? Skin temperature—this is not significant in the lab because you're on a warm water bed and everybody's hand temperature goes up. Pulse rate and galvanic skin response—I couldn't find much specific change there. But skin potential voltage, or polarity—what about that? I'd never measured it previously because I didn't think there was anything there. Then Bob Monroe told me to look at it, and I saw that as the skin potential voltage passed zero, going up or down, more often than not we would have a low-frequency power surge in the brain, which would trigger one of those escalating eddies or harmonics upward. Is it possible that there's a third measure, that as the skin polarity shifts so the brain has an opportunity to move into a transcendent state? We know it does when we go to sleep—it could be doing it otherwise.

We tested the participants in one Gateway program, before and after the program itself. There was a reduction in alpha density in all except one; they made less alpha. Was that because they had less vigilance or was it the effect of the program—or both? There was also much more higher-frequency activity, above 30 Hz in the right temporal lobe. Eighty percent were having temporal lobe activation at the end of the program.

Now we have a measure of penetrance here. You can measure

how many microvolts you get out of the temporal lobe when you stimulate the different frequencies (Focus 10, 12, 15, 21) and you can chart the actual power you are getting out of the temporal lobe as you are delivering these frequencies. After the program you see that the power delivered in the higher frequencies by the temporal lobe increases. When someone says "That's the one I get off on—I'm a Focus 15 person," you can see that they are producing a lot of power at a high frequency when they are getting the Focus 15 stimulus. We at last have a means of testing for the penetrance of the frequency following response of the person studied. The program change shows increased power, a higher order of Hemi-Sync signal over baseline levels at Focus 15 and 21; in other words, the person has learned something in the program, and you can demonstrate that learning in the brain waves, not only by what he says is going on.

I tested that against other means of entrainment. I created a tape using the Fibonacci series, and I could get low-frequency entrainment with it, whereas I got high-frequency entrainment with Hemi-Sync. That is a test for sensitivity to frequency stimulation in the brain.

What does this lead to? I have a theory that this is like Carl Jung's method of looking at the world—about the dimensions of attention. I think what we do with the Hemi-Sync process, and with other processes of healing and psychical activity, channeling and so on, is that we grease the transits of our knowing. Some of us stay stuck in our focus; we have a little domain in which we live, and we don't venture out of it because everything is strange and weird outside. Some of us are very narrowly focused, absorbed, living in this domain. Shifting to open focus may mean opening to a broader expanse of awareness. We know that the dimension of hearing, from low to high frequencies, increases as we go to a broader expanse of knowing. The visual field enlarges as a person gets into greater open focus. Sensory experience of the body also increases with open focus for most of us. Most of us are so used to feeling tension and pain that we have shut it off, and we do so at great expense because of the enormous amount of pleasurable sensory experience we exclude with that. One of the saddest things is that we shut ourselves down so that we can become more rational.

So what we are doing with the Monroe process may be greasing the transits to states of awareness that we have prohibited for ourselves because they were not natural or normal, or were not legitimated by mentors in life; but they were things we had to discover by ourselves and in ourselves as we continued to grow.

When we use this process we begin to heal diseases we have within, because diseases are largely the result of being stuck in our perception as to what is good or bad.

For example, what makes me react with cold hands, pounding heart, and escalating blood pressure is a perception of performance anxiety, a desire to do better, because Mama didn't give me the rewards I had earned unless I came home with all "As." So everything in life that was good, particularly being loved, became contingent on performance. Those processes of organization of sensory input that precede conscious awareness have been powerfully influenced by my early conditioning, my idea of who I was as a person. That led me to certain forms of stress response in my life. I would respond neuro-muscularly if the world was not a safe place but full of fear, or I would respond vascularly about perfection and performance and that sort of thing. Or I'd respond in my brain, as if I were spaced out, behaving weirdly as a response to stress, because grandma always acted crazily and jumped out of the window if things were bad—so why shouldn't I respond that way? Or I'd respond with my hormones when my feelings were shifted and I couldn't justify it. Remember how often you missed periods when you were under love-stress? In London in the V2 blitz, half the women stopped menstruating.

These are physical manifestations of this "stuckness" that we live in, when we are stuck in a way of knowing that is no longer adaptive for us. So what we need to do, whether with Hemi-Sync or some other process, is something we call "greasing transits" between states. We need to teach the ability not only to become passive and relaxed but to become tense, to become angry as well as loving, to learn to honor the dualities of our life and not hold on to any one part of the duality that we find ourselves in. As we mature and get stronger, we need to learn how to honor the dualities instead of clinging to one over the other. We are learning the ultimate maturation of human beings, whether by educational application, transcendent application, spiritual application, or healing. For healing occurs when we are able to shift freely back and forth between our dualities. Disease occurs when we get stuck in one way of knowing.

When people are really going into ecstatic experience, I've seen them go up to 120 to 150 microvolts activity as they start into this process. On the chart can be seen a beautiful eddy or wave form that flows upward as the individual opens. I don't think that's just transmuting the alpha. I think it's new energy that's been freed up, or that the individual has allowed to be free. The first time I saw this,

I thought the person probably had temporal-lobe seizure, and I continued to think that for some time because of the intensity of that response.

Remember that when we measure these things we are looking at only about a centimeter of cortex; we are not getting any information from the deeper structures. I have a sense that what you are seeing comes from a deep structure, perhaps the corpus callosum. My real sense is that we have so little used our feeling and our capacity for love and our capacity for great openness that parts of our brain which connect the temporal lobe with the cortex, the cavdate nucleus, are not very well developed functionally. When we start opening ourselves to deep states of awareness, with feeling instead of cognition, we begin to energize these areas, to open a new way of knowing. We have always thought that we can know only through our minds, and now we've come to the terrible knowledge that we don't know that way. We really know only through our feeling. And when the feeling opens and we really begin to experience that, we want to experience it more and more. We can never have enough. A path opens that we begin to follow; in terms of Jung, the path of our great journey, our search for the great Mother within all of us.

Each of us is dealing with our own heritage. Our stress-response style, our way of perceiving the world, our way of knowing are largely gleaned from parents (or maybe it's something we've brought in with us—I don't know). Perhaps the way we eat is virtually fixed and patterned after about age three, and the language our body uses to express who we are in the world, how we interrelate with other people, and our expectations of life are all built out of our heritage. Our ambitions, and therefore our frustrations, are all born out of our heritage. Perhaps it's time to begin to look at how fluid this process can be, not how rigid, and how much we can learn from this process, not only intellectually but emotionally. How warm the world is if we are warm and how smart the world is if we are smart, and how much we condition the reality that we're dancing in! That's what I really like about this place—it's a place where your reality can dance—free.

Explanation of terms:

Hz or hertz—number of cycles per second

Delta, theta, alpha, beta and gamma refer to brain-wave frequencies. A simplified non-technical explanation follows:

Delta: 0 to 4 Hz. Deep meditative states, deep non-dreaming sleep.

Theta: 4 to 8 Hz. Deep relaxation, deep meditative states, and sleep. Related to suggestibility, enhanced learning, healing, and consciousness exploration. Also associated with various dissociative experiences.

Alpha: 8 to 13 Hz. Generally produced with the eyes closed and the mind at rest. It is said to relate to the way the individual processes and interacts with the world he or she perceives.

Beta: 13 to 30 Hz. Conscious awareness, analytic, alert wakefulness. Related to the brain's sensory-motor areas.

Gamma: 30 to 50+ Hz. Related to mystical and transcendent experiences during meditation. May represent a loss of ego boundaries; a sense of merging with other people; a sense of universal knowing.

Much depends on the region of the brain where the particular frequency is recorded and on any associated frequencies.

Delta is dominant in early infancy and theta in children between two and five years old, while the others (alpha, beta, gamma) are dominant in adults.

Brain wave frequencies also have a pathological significance (gamma is associated with seizures, schizophrenia, and temporal-lobe epilepsy, for example).

Focus 10, 12, 15, 21 (see Introduction)

Microvolt: one-millionth of a volt.

The Fibonacci series is an arithmetical progression derived ultimately from Pythagoras and later applied by the Italian mathematician Leonardo of Pisa, also known as Fibonacci, in the thirteenth century. It works by addition as follows: 0+1=1; 1+1=2; 1+2=3; 2+3=5; 3+5=8; 5+8=13, and so on.

Access Channels, Turning Tides

Joan Faroughy

Some years ago, Joan Faroughy, now age fifty-five, living in Cambridge, England, suffered a severe stroke which affected mainly the left side of her body leaving her severely disabled, unable to use her left arm or leg. In 1990, she was introduced to Metamusic and the Stroke Recovery Series. She also listened to selected exercises from the H-PLUS series. Joan wrote various reports on her experience of Hemi-Sync and they are combined, entirely in her own words, in the following paragraphs.

End of January, 1991. After listening to a selection of the tapes for some weeks, very interesting images are appearing during meditation. A blown-up netting, star-like, making connections, light on light, gold and brilliant. A blue dot sometimes appears in the center. I try to plug in to this network and to connect my strong right-hand side to the weaker left-hand side.

Wheeling along the bumpy flagstones outside King's College, I tried to localize the sensation of each bump. I was trying to redraw my body map.

I now have a very strong feeling of turning tides and another way of looking at things, of being able to let go of what does not immediately come to hand/mind, knowing and believing that you have it at your fingertips in the essential moment. Strange how I seem to gain strength by giving strength.

If the changing ideas are giving energy to a changing path in life, this has to be the positive aspect of impermanence. . .(God willing). Also interesting is a kind of opening up, a freedom to discuss everything with everyone. With this freedom comes a sort of ease which helps to shape events as I dream them. Without intending to be arrogant, I have a feeling of being in lucid partnership with my destiny—no more the victim of "slings and arrows" even though I might be drawing the bow. . .

February. After listening to Metamusic *Modem* I felt I was either on the verge of understanding the Creation, or on the verge of creating a world which would put me away in a place where no-one would understand!

Access Channels (H-PLUS). *[The Access Channel is established by specific phased sound signals and enables communication to be transmitted to all levels of awareness, physical, mental and emotional.]* They can't be only the opening between head and arms and legs (who needs arms and legs anyway?) but have to be between you and me—and on to X and to Y and to Z, heart to heart, and eyeball to eyeball, nation to nation, and beyond. . .If we manage to really learn the lesson and tap into the greater access channels, this has got to be the most important method of communication of all time.

I have a strong feeling of a tidal wave. We have to know how to surf it and ride it, otherwise it will just sweep us away. *N'est-ce pas?*

Early March. Switching into the "Ten State," I looked at outstretched and spasmed fingers then, with closed eyes, gently curved them down.

May. After a long gap when the tidal wave temporarily ebbed, it is now returning to a strong but gentle flow. So many opportunities are coming this way and I'm given all the signs to turn them around and give opportunities to other people.

Motor (Stroke Recovery Tape 6). I have listened two or three times to this and from the very first time I had a sort of "pre-movement," a definite impulse in the affected side, especially in fingers, toes, and forearm. The whole leg is moving quite nicely now, and with the help of the tape the ankle is slightly moving. The affected knee feels as though it's moving, so strong is the impulse, and I can only know it isn't by placing the unaffected finger on it during the exercise.

I feel I'm gradually starting to work consciously with the sound patterns, i.e., working them down the body and into the extremities. At this point I'm aware of a network, an interlacing between right and left sides. There is definite movement in the left shoulder, calf, and leg on the affected side.

General (Stroke Recovery Tape 5). I found this at first to be very lengthy—a seemingly never-ending, monotonous passage. My irritation was exacerbated by the fact that I was uncomfortable in a wheelchair. The tape for me would be more helpful with verbal instruction. Perhaps we are too conditioned to musical sounds. I wonder if Jean-Michel Jarre is working in a similar way to Monroe—consciously or unconsciously.

June. Listening again to *Motor*, it is very clear that the effect is cumulative. The feeling of "pre-movement" or impulse becomes stronger and stronger. It's a feeling that the area is starting to remember its function. Woweeee! We need to structure more carefully both the use of tapes and putting into practice, together with recording the process.

Stroke Recovery *Speech A* (Tape 1). I should say that loss of speech was not my problem; on the contrary, words pour off my tongue. But when listening to this tape I really tried to place myself in that situation.

If you construct the word, feeling consonant by consonant, you can sense exactly how the sound will physically emerge. It's good there is no apparent word-association as this would detract from the word-making process. I liked the way the process is mapped out, e.g. in. . .ice. . .idea. . .idiom. I wonder whether you should promote the instruction of using the outbreath when saying the word. If this is a good idea, perhaps you should start off with aspirates "hoof. . .hollow. . .hello" as they are much easier to achieve than hard consonants and closed sounds. A small, realistic goal is a powerful motivator toward greater things.

An interesting observation since I've been working with the tapes is that I'm less and less aware of my disability. In fact, if I hold a brief image of myself, it's not one of a disabled person. Neither is it the person I used to be. Rather, the person that is. And this has given me the freedom to explore and to take risks, and to be curious about my possibilities—and to push back the boundaries and limits. There is so much more to come—it's almost alarming to be the vehicle. But travel I must, and probably give a ride to many on the way.

July. Physiotherapy at the hospital. For a while I've been wondering how the therapist can keep on slogging away without losing heart. It must be hard when she works so blooming hard not to see a result! Today there was the slight flicker of a response. Slight maybe, but response nevertheless. It is so important to have faith. Too many people have invested too much of theirs in me for me not to respond. This condition has helped me to forge so many links. The Access Channels are really forging ahead!

For me, the most important revelation was experiencing the Access Channels. Through contact with others on the path came the awareness of there being greater channels and lesser channels. I am blessed to be guided by the former and privileged to be occasionally regarded by some as the latter. Yet another insightful experience is that I do not have to regain my former physical condition in order to be myself and to be of service. That's not to say I accept my condition absolutely and entirely, but I no longer waste my time whilst awaiting the miracle.

February 1992. After re-reading my notes and observations, I realize I have completed the first loop of the spiral. With the aid of Hemi-Sync I feel that my personal growth and development are unfolding and following the same pattern as every spiral in nature. For this reason I would like to listen again to the tapes and record the experience anew. I feel sure that a second listening at this time would "hit deeper" and reach new terrain—terrain which should be charted and cultivated.

May 1992. Have listened frequently and at regular intervals to the tapes. I've realized the importance of not having expectations, but to let things unfold gradually.

After *General* and *Motor* came an increased awareness of self and of my affected arm and leg. The physical reactions were very strong, with an intense itching in palm and center sole (two points I am advised to treat with hot sesame oil and nutmeg by a doctor of traditional Tibetan medicine).

During physiotherapy sessions there is definite progress in both limbs. The therapists have noted more strength and control. And although my walk is still very much a stroke-pattern hobble, there is miniscule improvement.

I'm tending to work more with the "spiritual" part of myself. Perhaps being confined to a chair is what is necessary now. The Access Channels are widening, communication freely flowing.

After a period of doubt and confusion, the next phase has become crystal clear. It is to deepen my understanding of Buddhism and to develop the meditation practice. To clean up my body. To this end, I plan to spend time in Switzerland at a macrobiotic center and to participate in Level II of their program in the Ancient Healing arts.

Today the mists have cleared to reveal a clearly defined and sometimes tortuous mountain path.

Note. The Stroke Recovery series consists of six taped exercises designed to guide the listener in selecting collateral neural pathways and/or centers to replace those damaged or destroyed through stroke or traumatic head injuries. The exercises focus on the progressive recovery of speech and motor skills and on the facilitation of the general healing process.

The Path of Devotion: A Personal Story

Suzanne tells this story in her own words.

In 1977, I traveled to a remote, pristine wilderness area in Montana where, with thirty others, I participated in an intensive ten-day seminar to explore human consciousness and to learn to access meditative states. The seminar was one of The Monroe Institute's first structured programs and was attended by a wide cross section of people, including physicians, psychologists, artists, attorneys, writers, psychics, and actors, all interested in the creative process within expanded states of human consciousness.

This experience opened a door to inner exploration and discoveries that would continue for the rest of my life. I began thereafter to visit The Monroe Institute for seminars and experiential work in order to deepen and expand my knowledge and understanding of human consciousness.

In the following year, my younger sister was diagnosed with ALS (amyotropic lateral sclerosis, or Lou Gehrig's disease), and thus began for her, for her family, and for ours, an intensely confronting nine-year journey that would take her and all of us into a reality far beyond what any of us were prepared to observe or experience; where we would witness a process of human suffering that would rip the protective veils from our eyes and would burn holes in our hearts; where the boundaries between an unreal, insane world and ordinary reality would be shattered by living an experience so abhorrent to the senses and the spirit that the mind would be unable to contain it. Entering this reality would require us to be present to, to struggle against, to surrender to, a process beyond our control. We would learn to live in a time-extended moment between life and death, and to walk a precarious edge between hope and despair. ALS would be my sister's teacher. My sister would be our teacher.

Some five years later, I headed for the Institute to strengthen my own inner resources and also to see if I could uncover anything that could help my sister as her condition continued to grow worse. The disease process is one that very slowly traps a fully alert consciousness in a "dead" body; a death of the muscles and nerves of the entire body begins with a fatally creeping kind of quicksand paralysis so that by this time she was fully paralyzed from her feet to her neck but was still able to speak. Eventually she would be unable to move her lips and would communicate through eye movements. Finally, she would be unable to swallow, and she would die of starvation and thirst.

At the time I decided to make my visit, my sister's spirits and her spiritual strength (which throughout her ordeal had been astonishingly unshakable) had begun to slip away from her and she felt herself sinking into a hopelessness and a self-pity which she loathed. She wanted desperately, she said, to renew and strengthen her faith.

On the last evening of the seminar we were introduced to Focus 21, a new set of sound frequencies designed by Monroe to offer access to greater awareness and new levels of consciousness. As the tape was beginning, in a state of passionate and deep intent, I requested help from the highest intelligence in the universe available to me to assist me in helping my sister through this time. I continued the familiar preparatory process, gradually slipping deeper into the meditative state I had come to know so well. In this dimension of "no time, no space" it was impossible to discern how much time had passed when I became suddenly aware of a radiant, penetrating gold and white light, of intense warmth, together with the clear sense of a presence. Waves of convulsive-like movements rippled through my physical body. As the light grew brighter and more intense, I became surrounded by it, enveloped by it, and then, with what seemed like the explosion of a huge sunburst, my consciousness shattered into a million pieces and became one with the center of this brilliant and expanding light. With total knowing and complete clarity, I understood that I would be assisted. I knew that, even if I received no specific guidance about how to help my sister, my own reservoir of strength and love had been filled by this experience. I was encompassed by an overwhelming release of immense joy, of profound gratitude, accompanied by tears of appreciation. I *knew* then what cannot be put into words and this will remain with me the rest of my life.

I did not tell my sister I was going to ask for help for us. I did not want to get her hopes up and also I did not know what process would unfold once I arrived at the seminar. Often one's "plans" are preempted by the present moment and what seemed like a good idea before doesn't make any sense in the "Now" of today.

When I returned home, I called her. Her husband propped the telephone on a pillow next to her ear and mouth and left us alone to visit, which was our habit when I was not with her in person. After we had caught up on our family news, she said she wanted to tell me of an experience she had.

On the same evening that I had journeyed into Focus 21, she said she had moved into a most unusual state as she went to sleep. It seemed unclear to her whether it was a dream or whether it was real. She found herself outside the house, running up and down the mountain road surrounding their home. Her feet could actually feel the gravel on the road; she could feel her body moving through space, and the sensation of herself running, and I also recall she mentioned even seeing and touching flowers along the road. She described how filled with wonder and happiness she was to be outside, outdoors. She was thrilled with the sensation of movement and the sense of freedom she could feel in her body, and I could imagine how ecstatic she must have felt as she was cut loose and unshackled from her bed prison—excitedly, playfully running up and down the country road. Although she said that some part of her sensed this was "an experience" or dream, the profound awareness and sensation of running filled her with astonishment and joy. Moments later, she said, she was swooshing down a dark tunnel, which opened into a room where a group of people were gathered, all looking toward her as she catapulted in. She said it was so real that she was able to touch the wallpaper on the wall and feel its texture with her fingertips. A very kindly man standing in the center of the room said, "Ginny, we've been waiting for you. Welcome. We have something we think will help you. It is Bakti Yoga."

At this point, she said, her memory faded, but she expressed excitement, wonder, and curiosity about the experience.

Upon hearing my sister's story, I recounted my own experience to her and added that in my seminar at Monroe that week had been a mathematician scholar from Washington, D.C., who also happened to be a serious student of Yoga and very familiar with Eastern philosophy and practice. We both immediately wanted to contact this person, since neither of us had any knowledge of yogic literature nor had we ever heard of the term "Bakti."

In retrospect, although we were fully aware that a profound communication had occurred, we seemed to accept somehow that this kind of event was totally possible and even, in a way, ordinary.

It seems strange, looking back on our reaction, that we were not awestruck, but we seemed to be operating in a framework of "Well, of course this can happen!" We decided that I should call my mathematician friend at once and get to the bottom of this Bakti Yoga mystery.

When he answered, I excitedly poured out my story to him. Without a second's delay, he responded, "Yes, I know Bakti Yoga. It is the yoga of devotion—the path of devotion. The yoga discipline of devotion." Although we continued to talk, I can remember little because at the moment he told me what Bakti was, I was dumbstruck. Bakti Yoga—of course! What else for a human being to do who is utterly helpless to move her body and who feels her spiritual life eroding, who will not give in to despair yet desperately prays for a renewed nourishment of the soul?

I was stunned. The full awareness of what had happened—the fact that communication on such a level had occurred at all—the stunning clarity of the message and its seemingly perfect content—a path suggested to my sister, or confirmed, for restoring her spiritual existence, coupled with my own experience—all this hit like a bolt of lightning. Looking back, I think I wandered around for days in a state of profound wonder and gratitude; surely in a state of non-ordinary consciousness!

For my sister, although she did not take up the formal study of Bakti, the experience was a clear and powerful confirmation of her already well-traveled path of faith and devotion, an energizing force strengthening and bringing back to life a languishing spirit. She went on (and I mean to imply no causality here) to live for four more years during which, accompanied by her nurse and with her portable respirator strapped to her wheelchair, she attended her children's school events, community gatherings and celebrations, went on day trips to the ocean with her husband and, despite the ravagings of her disease, lived the active listener, supporter, mentor role of mother to her children.

When I was asked to share this experience in writing, I was not sure how clear the recall would be. But as I began to write, the vividness returned. I find, however, that I am unable—or perhaps hesitant—to label what happened, or to seek to "explain" or interpret it. Any attempt to conceptualize or categorize seems to desecrate it.

Easing the Way: A Personal Story

Stella is Jewish. Her parents were married in Cologne, Germany, early in 1933, at a time when tension and anxiety were high in Jewish neighborhoods and thousands of Jews were being rounded up and dispatched to "relocation camps" under the Hitler regime. As many of their relatives had already been taken to these camps, Stella's parents decided to emigrate to South Africa while they were still able to do so. There Stella was born. All her parents' relatives were exterminated in the Nazi death camps during the war. After the war ended, the family moved to the U.S.A. and began another life, this time as naturalized U.S. citizens.

Stella's mother had a medical history of constant illness and disease. She was diagnosed with Krohn's Disease, growths in the lungs, arthritis, and diverticulitis; finally, cancer claimed her in August 1991. Ever since leaving Germany she felt that she had deserted her family by seeking her own safety in South Africa to escape Nazi persecution. So, it seems, she made certain, through her many diseases and illnesses, that she suffered comparably to her relatives who died at the hands of the Nazis. Her entire life was spent trying to ascertain her own self-worth.

When Stella returned home from an Outreach workshop in August 1991, she discovered that her mother, now age seventy-eight and already receiving hospice care, had been taken seriously ill and was hovering between life and death. At the workshop she had heard the tape *Inner Journey* and had been very impressed by it. She took a copy to her mother's home and played it through a stereo player virtually non-stop for the next two days. Before the music began, her mother was restless and disturbed, but while it was playing she became more restful and at times was lucid enough to speak with members of her family. Throughout the two days she spoke of how she had been "visiting" with her own mother, who had been murdered during the Holocaust, and with other relations of hers who had also been killed. She was, it seemed, impelled to talk about these "visits," and at the same time she wanted to make her own transition but was finding it appallingly difficult to make the final decision to "let go."

Her family members were in a real dilemma as to what to do for the best. It was a Friday evening, just before the beginning of the Sabbath, and Stella decided to call the local Rabbi, who knew her mother, and asked him to stop by and say a prayer while she was in such a state of turmoil. He arrived soon and began to pray. As he did so, he became aware of the music playing in the background; it affected him emotionally and he began to cry, feeling very deeply the complexity of the situation. When he was leaving he asked Stella what the music was, saying that never before had he been so moved or filled with such deep emotion.

After the Rabbi left to conduct the evening service, the family gathered around Stella's mother, with *Inner Journey* still playing, praying and bidding her to turn to the white light and enjoy her time with her beloved relations who had made their transitions many years ago. She took a last breath, called out "Mama, I am here!" and let go of her physical life.

At the memorial service the Rabbi asked again about the music and Stella pressed the tape into his hand. She says that *Inner Journey* not only helped to keep her mother calm and serene as she made her final transition but also that it helped the family, the Rabbi and, perhaps most of all, herself, as she had been in continuous attendance on her mother during those last days and nights. Subsequently, whenever Stella hears that music it brings her mother closer to her and she finds the experience wonderfully uplifting.

Applications: Scientific and Technical

Chapter 7

Hemi-Sync and Electrocortical Activity

The study of consciousness, once seen as the poor cousin of the physical sciences, is rapidly becoming the center of attention in science.

Stansilav Grov, *M.D., The Holotropic Mind*

Research into hemispheric synchronization, the frequency following response, and other components of the Monroe process has intensified in the last few years. Laboratories in the United States and Canada are investigating the effects of Hemi-Sync on brain activity and the first results of their work are beginning to appear. Candidates for higher degrees are also submitting research into Hemi-Sync: two recent examples are Dale S. Foster's dissertation on the subjective and EEG correlates of Hemi-Sync for his Ph.D. at Memphis State University and Karen Varney's paper on the use of Metamusic as an adjunct to intervention with developmentally delayed children for her M.Ed. at Virginia Commonwealth University.

This chapter includes a ground-breaking report by Dr. M.R. Sadigh and Dr. P.W. Kozicky, of the Gateway Institute, Bethlehem, Pennsylvania, on the effects of Hemi-Sync on electrocortical activity and a technical report by Dr. Edgar Wilson on the relationship between Hemi-Sync and transcendent states of consciousness.

Further information on the scientific and technological aspects of Hemi-Sync may be obtained from The Monroe Institute.

The Effects of Hemi-Sync on Electrocortical Activity

M.R. Sadigh, Ph.D. and P.W. Kozicky, M.D.

Introduction

Bilateral hemispheric synchronization is a phenomenon that has been attracting the attention of researchers and clinicians for some time. It has been approximately thirty years since a number of studies showed that adept meditators tended to bring about a state of phasic hemispheric synchrony while in deep meditation (see Carrington, 1977). In a classic and oft-cited study, Banquet (1973) demonstrated that advanced TM meditators could indeed achieve total brain synchrony after a few minutes of repeating a mantra. However, even in adept meditators the dominant brain-wave frequency in which the state of synchrony occurs is almost impossible to predict and/or control.

Banquet suggested that during meditation a greater equalization of the functioning of the hemispheres tends to take place. This relative shift in hemispheric dominance (from left-brain dominance to whole-brain synchrony) may result in therapeutic effects which are likely to enhance mind-body integration and overall improvements in physical and emotional health. Because of a reduction in cognitive activities during moments of whole-brain synchrony, it is believed that negative thinking, self-punitive thoughts, and excessive worrying are apt to diminish and consequently a reduction in cognitive anxiety is experienced (Carrington, 1977; Schwartz, Davidson & Goleman, 1978; Sadigh, 1991).

Delmonte (1984) suggested that creative intelligence requires the synthesis and collaboration of both the analytic and the spatial/intuitive halves of the brain. Again, it appears that this left-brain/right-brain synthesis can be achieved almost at will by adept meditators, especially those who practice TM.

Green and Green (1989) believed that long-term biofeedback and relaxation training resulted in a harmonious relationship between the two hemispheres, which facilitated control of the autonomic nervous system. This control can be especially helpful in the treatment of a variety of stress-related and psychosomatic disorders. They also suggested that such states of bilateral synchrony may indeed bring out positive changes in psychophysical health, as well as therapeutic alterations in underlying personality characteristics which may interfere with healthy growth and development.

Ornstein and Thompson (1984) criticized the Western emphasis on intelligence in terms of the written or spoken word. They believed that possibly the reason we have difficulties expanding our standards of education is that we over-emphasize the potentials and abilities of the analytic/verbal brain. Studies investigating whole-brain synthesis clearly suggest that human knowledge, intelligence, and well-being may well flourish as the two brains begin to function as one—in unison and synchrony.

The following table summarizes some of the documented characteristics of the two hemispheres:

Left Brain	Right Brain
Verbal	Visual
Analytic	Perceptual
Cognitive	Affective
NREM Sleep	REM Sleep
Rational thinking	Intuitive

But how can we achieve whole-brain synchrony without needing to become involved in the prolonged practice of meditation and meditative exercises? Can such states be induced and maintained by the use of technology? To answer these questions, let us turn to the examination of Eastern and Western approaches which attempt to bring about whole-brain integration and synchrony.

From East To West: In Search of the Synchronized Brain

The beneficial effects of hemispheric synchrony suggested in the current literature have motivated a large number of researchers, clinicians, and entrepreneurs to discover more effective and practical ways of inducing such a state. Empirical research with some forms of meditative practices has shown that a synchronized brain state may be achieved but only after years of practice. Furthermore, it has been established that only certain forms of meditation result in such a state. Practices that require focused attention, such as TM, seem to be the most effective ways of causing whole-brain integration. As indicated earlier, synchrony achieved in this way appears to be limited to certain specific frequencies and states of consciousness which cannot be easily controlled or modified by the meditator.

A few years ago, we had the opportunity of mapping the cortical activity of an adept meditator who had been regularly practicing and teaching TM for some fifteen years. The subject's EEG activity during baseline showed an asynchronous state throughout the cortex. The primary cortical activity was that of high-frequency alpha, combined with some theta and beta waves especially concentrated in the left temporal lobe. Once a stable baseline was achieved, the subject was asked to begin his mantra meditation. Shortly afterwards, the subject's cortical activity began to slow down and signs of phasic-bilateral synchrony became apparent. Within a matter of minutes, the subject's primary cortical activity was that of low-frequency alpha across the cortex. This is consistent with similar observations reported in the literature (e.g., Basquet, 1973). After the subject ceased meditating, his cortical activity began to resemble that of the pre-meditation state.

This was the first time we witnessed a fully synchronized brain induced by meditation in our neuropsychological laboratory. The results and findings of this experiment were both exciting and sobering. "Do we need years of training in meditation before we can achieve whole-brain synchrony? If so, how many years?"

In the following months, by using our computer-analyzed EEG unit, we began testing and experimenting with a variety of equipment, gadgets, tapes, special vibrational sounds, and musical notes played on synthesizers, resonating bowls, and gongs, all of which were claimed to entrain the brain into a synchronized, enhanced state. The results were disappointing. In study after study, these devices and sounds failed to result in even a slight movement in the direction of hemispheric synchronization or enhancement of any brain-wave frequencies.

In the early months of 1989, we began studying the effects of a specialized audio technology known as Hemi-Sync, which purported to bring about hemispheric synchronization by inducing a frequency following response within the brain (Monroe, 1982). We designed three studies to measure and investigate the effects of the Hemi-Sync signals on electrocortical activities.

The First Pilot Study

Subject and Procedures

The first subject was a twenty-year-old right-handed white female. She volunteered to participate in the study. She had heard tapes carrying the Hemi-Sync signals in the past, although she said that she did not listen to such tapes on a regular basis. During the experiment, the subject was seated in a comfortable recliner in a dark room. Gold-plated EEG electrodes of a sixteen-channel grass EEG model 8-10c were attached using a modified "10-20" system electrode placement. The EEG unit was then interfaced with the HZI computer system for analysis and dynamic brain mapping.

Method

A simple, single-subject reversal design (ABA) was used in this study. In other words, the experiment consisted of three phases: the baseline (A); exposure to Hemi-Sync, or the treatment phase (B); and finally a post-treatment phase similar to the baseline phase (A). During the baseline phase, the subject's cortical activity was measured while she rested in the recliner. Once the baseline was established, the subject listened to a Hemi-Sync tape known as *Introduction to Focus 10*. The subject's EEG was again recorded during this phase. After completing the treatment phase, a post-treatment evaluation of the subject was made while she was merely resting.

Results

Close examination of the subject's baseline data showed an asynchronous mixture of alpha and beta activity (*Fig. 1*, p. 221). The beta activity was especially evident in the frontal lobes. During the treatment phase, however, the cortical activity was completely different. Full phasic hemispheric synchronization was observed across the cortex (*Fig. 2*, p. 221). The subject's primary brain activity was that of synchronized theta. The secondary activity was that of synchronized alpha. These results were quite astonishing since it is difficult to achieve and maintain a fully synchronized theta state. In the post-treatment phase, the subject's EEG activity began to resemble that of the baseline phase, with one exception: the frontal beta activity was completely absent. This possibly indicates that a normalization of cortical activity might have happened as a result of the Hemi-Sync exposure in the treatment phase. The significance of our findings from this study motivated us to design other similar studies.

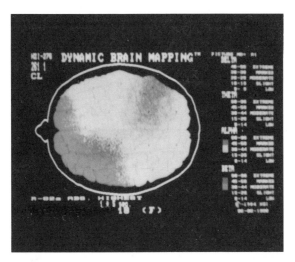

Figure 1.

Subject's electrocortical activity during the baseline phase. Asynchronous Alpha and Beta brain waves are present across the cortex.

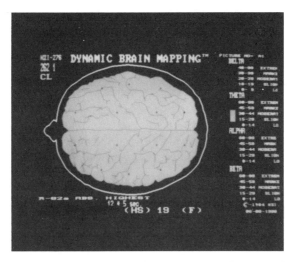

Figure 2.

Subject's electrocortical activity during the treatment phase (Focus 10). Full bilateral Theta synchrony is evident across the entire cortex.

The Second Hemi-Sync Study

Subject & Procedures

The subject was a forty-two-year-old right-handed white male, who volunteered to participate. He also had listened to Hemi-Sync in the past but indicated to us that he had not been practicing with such tapes for some time. The experimental procedures in this study were the same as in the previous study.

Method

A simple reversal design (ABA) was also used in this study. However the treatment phase (B) consisted of listening to a different Hemi-Sync tape, known as *Free Flow 12*. This and the *Focus 10* tape are standard exercise tapes that are available through The Monroe Institute.

Results

During the baseline phase, the subject's cortical activity consisted of asynchronous theta and alpha waves. However, a few minutes after the subject began listening to the *Focus 12* tape, his cortical activity began to show bilateral synchronous beta waves (*Figs. 3 & 4,* page 223.). The subject was able to maintain such "high power" synchronized state while he was listening to the tape. The remarkable shift in brain-wave patterns and the phasic synchrony which was induced by the Hemi-Sync signal can be appreciated by examining the stripchart recordings made during the session (*Fig. 5,* page 224). The induction of such a hyper-synchronous state by means of audio signals is unique and unheard of in the literature.

The subject's cortical activity returned to an asynchronous but more normalized state during the post-treatment phase. Because of the significant findings of this study we decided to replicate it at a later date.

The Third Hemi-Sync Study

In our third study we replicated every condition, procedure and methodology used in the second study. Again, the same subject's brain-wave activity was recorded during the baseline phase (A). He then listened to the *Focus 12* tape while his cortical activity was monitored and recorded (B). Finally, the subject rested while post-treatment recordings were made (A).

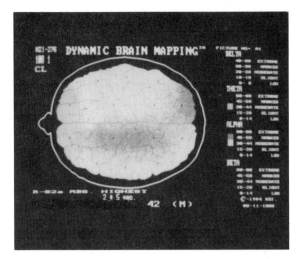

Figure 3.

Subject's electrocortical activity during the baseline phase. Asynchronous Alpha and Theta brain waves are present across the cortex, as arrows indicate.

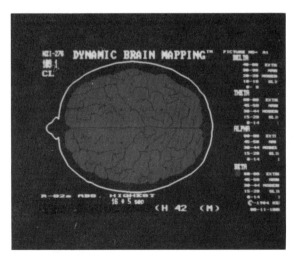

Figure 4.

Subject's electrocortical activity during the treatment phase (Focus 12). Full bilateral Beta synchrony is evident across the entire cortex.

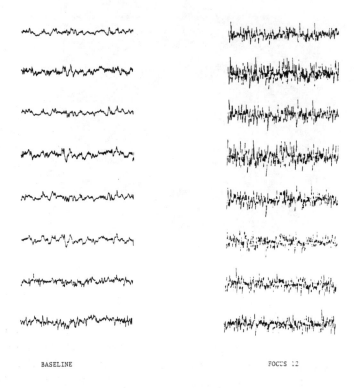

BASELINE   FOCUS 12

Figure 5.

The results and findings of this study were virtually identical to those observed in the second study: asynchronous mixture of theta and alpha waves during the baseline phase, followed by highly synchronized beta activity across the cortex during the treatment phase. The only difference was that it took the subject even less time to produce synchronized brain waves. This may indicate that the more an individual is exposed to Hemi-Sync, the easier it will be for him/her to achieve whole-brain integration.

Discussion & Conclusions

It has been documented that probably all of us experience very brief moments of bilateral phasic hemispheric synchronization every day. However, this phenomenon is outside the control of the great majority. Even those adept meditators who appear to induce such a state while meditating do not seem to have any control over the brain-wave frequency at which this synchronization occurs. Furthermore, it may take many years before a serious meditator can achieve full cortical synchrony. Even after years of practice there are, of course, no guarantees that one may experience this unique phenomenon.

Because of the beneficial and therapeutic effects of whole-brain integration, numerous types of equipment, recorded sounds, and various technologies are now available which promise and claim to induce such a state. However, based on our empirical studies, we have found that none of these approaches seems able even to entrain the brain toward a state of synchrony. Thus far, we have been able to document that the only effective technology that results in bilateral hemispheric synchronization is the Hemi-Sync technology developed by Robert A. Monroe.

In study after study we have been able to demonstrate that, after brief periods of exposure to Hemi-Sync signals, subjects' brains began to enter into a state of phasic synchrony. This state appears to be similar to what is experienced cortically by some meditators, with the following exceptions. First, unlike meditation, Hemi-Sync does not require years of practice. We have been able to demonstrate in our laboratory that after only a few minutes of exposure to the signal full cortical synchrony is achieved. Second, while the hemispheric synchrony experienced during meditation appears to be limited to a certain range of brain-wave frequencies, Hemi-Sync appears to induce a variety of synchronized states at almost any frequency. In other words, the Hemi-Sync signal is capable of facilitating a variety of states of consciousness ranging from deep sleep to focused concentration and beyond. Finally, we have observed that after periods of exposure to the Hemi-Sync signal a phenomenon of cortical normalization tends to occur. This beneficial effect seems to be unique to Hemi-Sync, since we have not observed anything similar to this with our meditation subjects.

Since we first demonstrated that Hemi-Sync does indeed do what it purports to do, we have continued our experiments with this fascinating brain-entrainment modality. We are now documenting some of the beneficial effects, both emotional and cognitive, that are induced as a results of moments of comparatively brief exposure to Hemi-Sync (see Sadigh, 1991). Studies with larger samples are now needed in order to investigate individual differences and how Hemi-Sync may affect specific brain-wave activities in different individuals.

225

References

Banquet, J.P. (1973). "Spectral analysis of the EEG in meditation." *Electroencephalography and Clinical Neurophysiology*, 35, 143-151.

Carrington, P. (1977). *Freedom in Meditation.* New York: Doubleday.

Green, E., and A. Green (1989). *Beyond Biofeedback.* New York: Delacorte Press.

Monroe, R.A. (1982). *The Hemi-Sync Process.* Unpublished MS, The Monroe Institute.

Ornstein, R., and R.F. Thompson (1984). *The Amazing Brain.* Boston: Houghton Mifflin.

Sadigh, M.R. (1991). "Hemi-Sync and Insight-Oriented Psychotherapy." *Hemi-Sync Journal*, 9, 1-2. (See Page 176 above.)

Schwartz, G.E., R.J. Davidson, and D.T. Goleman (1978). "Patterning of Cognitive and Somatic Processes in the Regulation of Anxiety: Effects of Meditation Versus Exercise. *Psychosomatic Medicine*, 40, 321-328.

A Technical Report
Edgar S. Wilson, M.D.

An independent psychophysiological study of the Hemi-Sync process was conducted by the Colorado Association for Psychophysiologic Research in October 1991. The purpose of the study was to determine whether the technique could enhance the induction of a transcendent experience. One male and two female adept subjects (experienced users of Hemi-Sync) were studied and compared with one male and two female naive subjects (who had little or no experience of Hemi-Sync prior to the beginning of the study). All subjects were examined while listening to the same series of sounds through stereo headphones, while lying supine in an isolated, shielded environment. The naive subjects were retested after attending the Gateway Voyage training seminar.

All subjects were connected to a twenty-channel, computerized EEG (Neurosearch-24). Data was collected at baseline (without sound), during stimulation with pink noise, and during each of four binaural beat frequency combinations delivered in sequence and embedded in pink noise. Subjective reports of the content of what was experienced were obtained during a debriefing session at the end of each experiment.

Data Analysis

Raw data was screened for artifacts and all epochs with over 80 uV spikes, indicating muscle artifacts, in any channel were discarded from analysis. The EEG data was scanned in raw form, and computation of averaged FFT (Fast Fourier Transform) of 50 epochs was computed at the end of each experiment. Color topograms were derived from each FFT histogram and compared for changes. Specific channels showing the greatest change were subjected to time-series analysis of band widths, ranging from delta frequencies to 64 Hz. "Burst" phenomena—high amplitude spontaneous EEG activity—were subjected to cascade analysis to determine their duration, power, frequency, and harmonic progression.

Results

Significant alterations in EEG frequency and power at the temporal lobes (T3 and T4) in females and at the median of the central cortex (CZ) in males were observed in both the adept and the trained naive subjects. Ascending bursts of frequencies as high as 64 Hz occurred in the temporal lobes in adept females. Males showed smaller incremental changes at the central cortex median. Adept subjects showed lower theta and alpha power-burst phenomena but higher frequency activity as the stimulus progressed.

Prior to attending the Gateway Voyage, the naive subjects showed similar responses to the first and second binaural beat stimuli (Focus 10 and Focus 12 in the Monroe terminology), but failed to show higher frequency entrainment to the third and fourth binaural beat stimuli (Focus 15 and Focus 21). When the naive subjects were retested after attending the training seminar, their performance levels approached those of the adept subjects.

A flowing, dynamic pattern of EEG activity accompanied the transcendent experiences reported by the subjects. At baseline and during stimulation with pink noise, alpha activity was confined to the cortex behind the Sylvian sulcus (*see Fig. 1*). As the stimulation progressed into the first two sets of binaural beat frequency mixes, this predominant alpha activity decreased somewhat and the subjects' EEGs began to show delta and theta activity at the central cortex (*see Fig. 2*). As the stimulation continued into the third and fourth sets of binaural beat frequency mixes, marked correspondence between low-frequency bursts within the auditory cortex could be seen to amplify in power at the CZ electrode followed by a progression to higher power and frequency (beta and gamma) activity in both adept and trained naive subjects. Beta and gamma activity in the median central cortex was typical of the males, while beta and gamma activity in the temporal lobes was characteristic of the females (*see Fig. 3*).

The subjective reports of the remembered content of state changes varied considerably among all subjects studied. No adverse or "bad" experiences were noted. Those showing higher-frequency EEG entrainment above the beta range more often reported "ecstatic" or "out-of-body" experiences. Lower-frequency responders often experienced sleep-like states with occasional vivid dreams.

Figure 1.

Alpha activity in the baseline phase. The lighter the shading, the greater the activity.

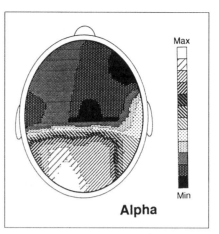

Alpha

Figure 2.

Delta/theta activity during the first two stages of binaural beat stimulation, showing the strongest activity at the central cortex.

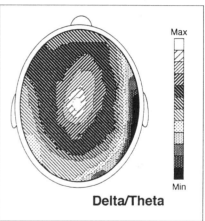

Delta/Theta

Figure 3.

Beta/gamma activity during the third and fourth stages, most marked in the temporal lobes—characteristic of females.

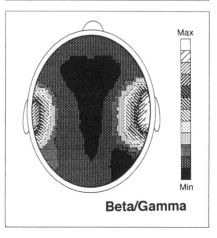

Beta/Gamma

Conclusions

Binaural beat auditory stimulation, as presented in the Monroe Hemi-Sync process, appears to provoke progressive entrainment or penetrance of EEG activity toward higher frequencies and specific patterns of "burst" phenomena. A comparison of naive subjects before and after the Gateway Voyage training program with known adept subjects suggests that a learning curve of progressive higher frequency sensitivity may be established. The commonalities of experiential reports during the Hemi-Sync training process may reflect preconditioning of the belief systems of the participants and/or a true progression of transcendent experience.

A similar study utilizing a different rationale is planned to determine if this auditory binaural beat technology and assessment method might be used to quantify more accurately progressive transcendent states of consciousness. The Hemi-Sync process, therefore, may provide a more controlled method of studying the psychophysiologic concomitants of progressive transcendent states of consciousness.

Note: On the scientific and technical aspects of the Hemi-Sync process, various research papers by F. Holmes Atwater, Administrator of Research, are available from The Monroe Institute. They include the following:

> The Monroe Institute's Hemi-Sync Process: A Theoretical Perspective
> EEG Brain Mapping of the Hemi-Sync Process
> EEG Alpha Density
> Gaining Access to Propitious States of Consciousness with the Hemi-Sync Process

Chapter 8

Domestic Animals

There seems no reason why animals—domestic animals especially—should not respond to Hemi-Sync. Some pets certainly do. When Dr. Suzanne Morris's dog was injured in an accident and needed to be kept quiet and relaxed so that he would not interfere with his bandages or try to do too much before his leg was healed, she settled him comfortably with headphones close by and played him Metamusic tapes for hours on end. Cheryl Williams used H-PLUS exercises to help heal her cocker spaniel, and Suki, the Russell Centre cat, often meditates to the strains of *Sunset* or *Midsummer Night.*

The first scientific study, however, was on horses in a series of experiments conducted by Dr. Helene Guttman.

A Hemispherically Synchronized Horse
Helene N. Guttman, Ph.D.

Dr. Helene Guttman has graduate degrees in three different branches of science. She currently holds a senior position in the Research Agency of the U.S. Department of Agriculture. Dr. Guttman has a special interest in biomedical areas and has published several papers on brain peptides that influence behavior.

Virtually all documented studies on the use of sound to modify behavior have been done using human subjects. These studies include a wealth of biomedical reports in the scientific literature and many others published in magazines and books aimed at a more general audience. One purpose of the process that has become known as Hemi-Sync is to utilize special binaural sound beats as a combination switch and entrainment signal that alerts both halves (hemispheres) of the brain to operate simultaneously for a particular task, whether it is relaxation, concentration, or whatever. When working with human subjects, one usually gathers oral, subjective reports from the subject during or after the experience. Sometimes it is useful to attach the subject to equipment that measures physiological reactions to determine whether subjective reports correlate with one or more physiological patterns.

Among farmers in many countries, it is common to play radio or tape-recorded music in barns, both to entertain the workers and, it is claimed, to keep the animals happy and productive. Reports in the European scientific literature indicate that noxious noises—noise pollution—appear to have negative effects on animals; for example, reduction in milk production or increase in levels of the so-called stress hormones. There are no reports of controlled experiments attempting to correlate changes in patterns of animals' brain waves with the onset or cessation of sound stimuli.

This study was the first step in determining if animals, other than humans, respond to Hemi-Sync signals by synchronizing the electroencephalographic (EEG) output of the left and right sides of their brains. More specifically, do horses (our chosen test species) respond to these signals with brain synchronization, and, if so, can we achieve this using inexpensive, non-invasive, portable (battery-operated) equipment that would not interfere with an animal's normal habits and behavior?

To answer this question, we administered two types of prerecorded sounds to a horse: (1) a control tape without Hemi-Sync sounds, and (2) an experimental tape that sounds the same as the control but has Hemi-Sync signals embedded under the control sounds. We selected music that the horse appeared to like, based on our observations of her responses.

It is important to eliminate the possibility that an investigator will obtain the desired results by inserting cues as to what he intends to happen. For example, some years ago primary school psychology experiments showed that telling teachers to expect certain groups of children to do well or poorly prior to the initiation of a teaching experience influenced the teachers to give, without realizing it, different amounts of attention to the different groups. The result was that the children said to be good learners did well, while those said not to be did poorly. The teachers unconsciously created a self-fulfilling prophecy.

The same sort of self-fulfilling prophecy can influence results in experiments in which animals are subjects if the investigator has not been "blinded" with regard to result expectations. The now classical report on maze learning in rats (Markowitz and Sorrells, Jr., 1969) is particularly useful as guidance for proposed studies involving Hemi-Sync effects on animals. Markowitz and Sorrells divided a litter of inbred rats into two groups and gave the groups to an investigator who was told that one group was derived from a line of slow learners and the other from a line of fast learners. The result was that rats from the supposedly fast-learning group performed well, while rats from the other group performed poorly—another self-fulfilling prophecy. These results emphasize the importance of coding treatments and keeping the investigator who is in contact with the subjects ignorant of any result expectations.

Either headphones or stereo speakers may be used for exposing animals to the music tapes. For these first experiments we used a stereo tape player. In subsequent experiments we used headphones. When headphones are used, it is important to position them at least an inch from the horse's ears, because horses do not like their ears to be touched. We used a music tape specially composed to fit the tempo of fifty to seventy beats per minute with a regular rhythm; this has been found to promote relaxation and enhance learning and retention skills in humans. The Hemi-Sync signals were embedded under the music so that we human experimenters could not hear the difference between the control tape and the Hemi-Sync tape. Both tapes were coded and the key to the codes was not given to me until the experiment was completed.

In his theoretical perspective of the Hemi-Sync process, Atwater (see Chapter 7) noted that the frequencies at which binaural beats can be detected change depending on the size of the cranium, and that the distance between the ears influences how the brain perceives the signal. Horses, compared with humans, have much bigger heads and thicker skulls, but have much smaller brains—about the size of a grapefruit.

These first experiments were geared only to determine whether we could find conditions that would result in synchronizing the brains of horses. Each experiment session took forty-five minutes. All experiments were recorded on videotape with the time and date marked on each frame and the sound track active. The subject horse was fitted with a battery-operated, simplified four-channel EEG (HAL-4) modified so that it could store the data on a buffer device and also be turned on and off remotely. The entire equipment apparatus was packed into a plastic carrying case that was strapped to the horse where the saddle ordinarily would go. The electrodes were secured to a card fixed with Velcro to a horse bonnet. Electrical contact with the horse's head was assured for each electrode by first clipping the forehead hair over the brain location and coating the electrode contact sites with electrical conducting jelly. The electrodes were connected to the modified HAL-4 by cables.

After the experiments were concluded, the data was downloaded from the buffer and stored on computer floppy disks for later analysis. This analysis consisted of using the HAL-4 software program to convert the EEG squiggles into an equivalent series of changing bar graphs, using the mathematical process known as Fourier transform. The bar graphs were displayed in such a fashion that we could see simultaneously on a computer graphic presentation the graphs made from the EEGs for both sides of the horse's brain. This enabled us to have a visual presentation over the range of brain frequencies, 4 to 20 Hz, that we monitored during the experiments, and to see if stimulus with Hemi-Sync signals that synchronized brains of humans also synchronized the brain of our horse. Typical pictures of the horse's unsynchronized brain patterns are shown in Figure 1. Typical pictures of synchronized horse brain patterns are shown in Figure 2.

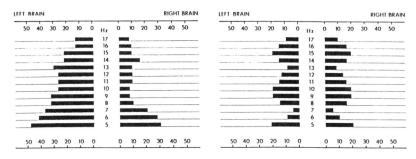

Left: Unsynchronized brain patterns of horse. Right: Synchronized brain patterns of horse while listening to Hemi-Sync tape signals.

This is then the first evidence that the same types of Hemi-Sync signals that synchronize the brains of humans also synchronize horse brains. This suggests various future uses for Hemi-Sync with equines, including (a) stress reduction during travel; (b) calming followed by attentiveness and alertness before races and horse shows; (c) enhancement of sleep and rest periods; and (d) environmental enrichment in their quarters. The use of brain monitoring is, of course, ancillary to the important visible behavioral effects of Hemi-Sync on humans and animals. Nevertheless, such monitoring is a research tool that assists us in understanding the mechanism of the underlying events.

It is worth noting that the subject horse, whose name is Some Match, showed no distaste for the experiments. She tolerated them willingly and indeed at times appeared to be enjoying what was happening.

A follow-up study with another horse, Kerry Mist, was recorded on videotape. The musical composition *Inner Journey* was used in two versions, one with and one without the Hemi-Sync signals, played through headphones incorporated in a specially designed hood which the horse had become accustomed to wearing.

Before the study began, Kerry Mist was quite calm and not troubled by the free-roaming stable mate in the pasture. Immediately before the tape was played, she exhibited the classic equine "relax stance" (one back leg raised and relaxed). The stable mate, Bonny Dick, came close and remained about one foot away facing her tail for the duration of the study.

During the playing of the non-Hemi-Sync tape, Kerry Mist maintained the "relax stance" and stayed alert to the music, as evidenced by orienting her ears toward the sound from the headphones. The weather was becoming uncomfortably hot and thunder began to rumble. Neither horse seemed startled by the thunder and they made no attempt to seek shelter. They remained still while the tapes were changed.

Listening to the Hemi-Sync tape, Kerry Mist maintained her "ears alert" position. She became progressively more relaxed, as evidenced by her head moving gradually lower until it was no more than twelve inches from the ground. Her manner became calmer and more detached from the surroundings, shown by the following observations: she did not swat the many flies that landed on her; her legs were no longer directly under her trunk so that she was no longer standing straight; she did not tug on her rope to signal she would prefer to move elsewhere (as she usually would with an approaching storm).

Kerry Mist maintained this demeanor until the tape was turned off and the hood and equipment removed. She then moved very slowly and lackadaisically, but without staggering, and remained in the pasture only a few feet from where she had been listening to the tapes. Finally she gave a succession of six big yawns. This horse had never before been seen to make serial yawns.

These results indicate that the addition of a theta-delta Hemi-Sync program to a free-flowing musical composition produces additional easily visible behavioral effects.

Horses become recumbent in only about three hours out of each twenty-four, and exhibit REM sleep only during recumbency. They are usually recumbent at night, and the state is preceded by relaxation and head lowering until it touches the ground. Since Kerry Mist had never before been observed to move into an almost recumbent state during a hot, humid day with a rapidly approaching electrical storm, it seems likely that this was induced by the combination of the music plus the embedded signals. This invoking of behavioral change in a horse suggests the potential of numerous uses for various Hemi-Sync embedded tapes with animals, including relaxing animals during transportation (usually a stressful procedure); inducing a state of relax-alert before tasks; and utilizing concentration tapes for training animals that are hyperactive and have difficulties learning new tasks.

The observation that Kerry Mist's stable mate stayed close to her during the whole of the tape episode suggests it would be interesting to follow the EEG output of close pairs ("friends") of animals (including humans) to determine whether the EEG output in the member not receiving direct audio stimulation changes to resemble the EEG output of the subject. In addition, future experiments now in the planning stage will investigate pigs and also interspecies relationships; for example, those between Border Collies and the sheep they herd.

Outreach

Chapter 9

Outreach Programs

The Outreach program was introduced in 1985 to meet the many requests for Hemi-Sync training close to home. The first of the program's components is the Excursion workshop, a two-day adventure, normally residential, into the expansion of consciousness by gentle increments so that states of profound relaxation, deep contemplation, and communication with the total self—and perhaps with non-physical energies—may be experienced. Specifically designed tapes with the Hemi-Sync technology form the core of the program, together with explanation, discussion and supportive group interaction.

More recently, the two-day H-PLUS workshop was introduced. This workshop enables greater personal control over mental, emotional, and physical well-being. It teaches skills for relaxation, concentration, memory, pain control, maintenance of physical health, creativity, release of negative emotion, and more. The emphasis is on learning practical tools to use in daily life.

These workshops, along with others specially designed to provide Hemi-Sync support for a wide variety of interests and personal goals, all conducted by accredited trainers, are available throughout the United States and in many other countries. Selected tapes have been translated into several European languages. This chapter includes accounts by four of these trainers describing the work that they do.

Excursion Training

Judith Taylor

Judith Taylor runs Excursion training in Montville, New Jersey. Her participants range in age between the mid-twenties and the sixties, the ratio of men to women being 45% to 55%. Engineering is the profession most represented, with data analysts next. Other occupations include physicians, psychologists, educators, lawyers, carpenters, management consultants, salespersons, maintenance mechanics, nurses, and psychic healers.

The reasons given for first attending a workshop include accessing one's "higher self," curiosity about the process, exploration of the out-of-body state, improving meditation techniques, and reprogramming one's daily life. The depth of the experience varies greatly, depending on the individual. It seems that the fewer expectations the participant has, the more likely he or she is to go to profound levels of awareness. The biggest stumbling blocks seem to be a rigid idea of what an experience should be and an over-eagerness to "get there." That the experiences are valuable, however, is evidenced by the fact that most participants have continued to use the exercises in their everyday life. Several have since taken residential courses at The Monroe Institute.

For most participants, the program seems to have sustained effects, including better dream recall, more lucid dreaming, increased physical energy, less need for sleep and shorter sleep cycles, improved concentration and recall, new awareness of subtle energies, increased incidence of psychic phenomena, and an improved ability to obtain insight into everyday problems. Perhaps the most universally expressed feeling in each workshop was the joy of being with a group of people who were all mentally and spiritually moving in the same direction—if only for two short days.

Discussion time after each tape is especially important, and participants often share quite dramatic—or traumatic—experiences with the group. Several have contacted deceased relatives and, in some cases, resolved issues that had not formerly been addressed. One had never grieved over the death of her father fifteen years before. In between two exercises she suddenly complained of chest pain. Her overall demeanor seemed healthy, and she considered that the symptom might relate to something the tapes were stirring up, although she had no idea what it was. During the next tape she made the connection: her father had died of a heart attack. It was during this tape that she felt she had finally completed her grief work.

Another participant, who was overweight and had tried unsuccessfully to slim down, also used a physical symptom as a vehicle for insight. In the middle of the tape, her body began to hurt. She went into the pain, allowing her awareness to be one with the pain, and was taken to a traumatic event when she was a teenager that had involved the left side of her body. This event appeared to her to be responsible for why she was overweight today. This realization gave her a new understanding of her present condition.

Several participants gained insight into practical problems in their everyday life, while most experienced, some for the first time, the exhilaration of being pure thought, unencumbered by the physical body. A few had full-blown out-of-body experiences, where they felt their consciousness leave their bodies and they were able to view the entire room from above. Others simply felt as if they were floating in a blissful state. Many complained vociferously about having to return to the normal conscious state when the exercise was over.

Two particular experiences were especially moving. One involved a woman who had been unable to have children. She was unexpectedly taken into a profoundly emotional past-life experience, where the reason for her current situation was explained to her. Although she had seemed to have adjusted to not having children, this experience gave her a deeper perspective on the situation.

The second experience concerned a songwriter who was convinced that he had lost his creativity after giving up cocaine. During the workshop he had a powerful out-of-body experience. Several days later he awoke in the middle of the night, having composed a song in his sleep. He began doing this on a regular basis, and some months later he returned to serious composing from a level of creativity he thought he would never experience again.

The most detailed example I can provide regarding the practical value of the Hemi-Sync process is my own. I was terrified of public speaking throughout my life and avoided it at all costs. The few times I had to speak, my voice would either crack noticeably or disappear altogether. Yet being a trainer necessitated that I speak for variously sized audiences and sometimes for quite a long time, either in the workshops or in the lectures I give to promote the technology and the process.

Hemi-Sync helped me to overcome this incapacitating fear in two ways. The meditation tapes enabled me to focus my attention on a lot of formerly unconscious material that was crippling me. I was eventually able to eliminate these self-defeating concepts. The H-PLUS *Speak Up* tape helped me to re-program myself mentally, so that I was not only able to speak clearly and smoothly but could also relax enough to do so from an expanded level of awareness. Most important is that I began to enjoy speaking to groups. Some of the enjoyment may come from my fascination with the technology and the miracles it can produce. Ultimately, I derive great pleasure from being able to facilitate for others some of the highly beneficial effects of Hemi-Sync through these workshops.

The Russell Centre

Jill and Ronald Russell

Jill and Ronald Russell co-direct the Russell Centre in Cambridge, England, and have been running courses and workshops using Hemi-Sync for over five years. England has a strong tradition of evening classes for adults, so they began by designing a sequence of evening sessions to cover similar ground to the residential weekends. A series of one- and two-day workshops was developed in addition, and six of these are now included in their program, three dealing progressively with personal growth and the others covering the H-PLUS series, healing, and out-of-body work. There are also "reunion evenings" for workshop participants.

When we first decided to run Hemi-Sync courses in England, we asked Robert Monroe what we should do to attract participants. His reply was, "Nothing—they'll come." And they have. Out of the hundred or so workshops we have run since we started, no more than three or four have had to be rearranged because of shortage of numbers.

In the beginning, participants were from Cambridge and the surrounding area but, somehow or other, the word soon spread. Inquiries came from London, fifty miles away; then from places like Wolverhampton, York, Warwick, and Dorset, up to two hundred miles distant. The circle continues to expand. We also travel to present workshops for particular groups, including hospital staffs.

Our policy included two specific points: to make participants as comfortable as possible and to keep costs as low as we could. One large room was cleared of furniture, close carpeted in wool, and equipped with a good sound system. We can take up to ten people, each on headphones with their own volume control. Another policy point was that we would share the workshops with the participants so that we remain with them all the time, listening to the tapes along with them. This group work produces its own dynamic; it brings everyone closer together and enables experiences to be more readily shared and exchanged.

Several teachers and nurses come to the workshops, as well as therapists of various kinds, businessmen and women, academics, and an increasing number of young scientists (but few older ones!). Having begun with the Introductory Workshop, almost all return for more and there are now several who have done everything that we can offer. Many use Hemi-Sync in their own lives and work, and a number have traveled to Virginia for courses at the Institute.

Compared to the inhabitants of the United States and some European countries, English people tend to be cautious or even skeptical when presented with something new. This is not necessarily a disadvantage; it means that the product or technique, whether Hemi-Sync or anything else, is examined critically and subjected to close scrutiny before being accepted. That Hemi-Sync stands up to this is very much in its favor.

To evaluate what we do, we rely greatly on feedback from participants. Comments that have been received include the following:

"I've been able to relax more and sleep whenever I want to."

"I'm feeling more in control of myself. I'm feeling more at one with others."

"[The tapes] help in achieving a positive attitude to various aspects of life. I feel more in tune with myself and with things—and also with other people."

"I've found a decrease in the severity and frequency of migraine attacks. I feel more relaxed—less prone to stress."

"Made giving up smoking easier. I'm now working at a slower pace."

"Many facets of my childhood have returned. This year in spring I noticed bird song for the first time for years. The deep, powerful enjoyment of literature has returned. I have felt less vulnerable, more confident. Practically speaking, I am sure I will soon pass my driving test." [She did.]

"I find the tapes are useful in times of stress or feeling low when, nevertheless, activity and commitment must continue in the normal way."

"I note the ability to be at ease with myself, understanding changes in me and around me. Also being able to cope with most things, especially at stressful times. Using my own energy to give me more energy. Being able to help others by being more patient and tolerant—understanding their weaknesses. Also not being afraid—not anything specific, just thoughts, death, etc. I feel more alive and positive, stronger and more capable."

Much of the value of a workshop lies in the discussion that takes place between the tape sessions. It is remarkable how quickly the tapes can break down the barriers, especially where the characteristically "reserved" English are concerned, and how lasting friendships between participants are often formed.

In addition to courses and workshops, we do a certain amount of individual work, mainly in the areas of sleep, anxiety, and pain control. Tapes which have proved especially useful include the *Pain Control* tape, H-PLUS exercises *Restorative Sleep*, *Let Go*, *Relax*, *Off-Loading*, and *De-Discomfort*, the *Concentration* tape and Metamusic *Inner Journey* and *Midsummer Night*. For relaxation, *Introduction to Focus 10* is extremely helpful. And, in spite of its title which calls to mind a garage mechanic's workbench, H-PLUS *Brain: Repair & Maintenance* is in frequent demand!

Seminars in Eastern Europe

Robert Siciliano

In 1991, when he was living in Germany, Robert (Kala) Siciliano embarked on a program to take the Hemi-Sync technology into Eastern Europe.

My experience of introducing the people of Poland, Hungary, and Czechoslovakia to the Hemi-Sync technology is especially interesting in that, although they have lived the better part of the last fifty years under intense suppression and have been depressed both emotionally and economically, I find them open, eager, and very willing to know what more is possible beyond what they already know in life. This includes the willingness to pay the small tuition fee required for attendance at the seminar, in order to cover expenses incurred in making my visit and the seminar possible, or to buy a Hemi-Sync tape. In most cases these costs exceed their monthly incomes. This makes the wanting to know and willingness to explore so obvious that it almost overwhelms me. I must say that this experience is rarely found in the more affluent West.

The seminar I present lasts for two and a half days and is a modification of the Excursion format, which presents the preparatory tools, an introduction to the Focus 10 state of "mind awake/body asleep," and to the Focus 12 state of expanded awareness, as well as the "release/recharge" exercise. All communication is via simultaneous translation of my instructions through a native interpreter. Participants lie on the floor while the tapes are played through open stereo speakers. I mostly use a specially designed nonverbal free-flow tape during the seminar.

The seminar begins on a Friday evening with an introduction explaining the technology. Then I play an introductory demonstration tape and deal with a question-and-answer session. A briefing of the program for the next two days comes next, which involves introducing the preparatory process and an explanation of the exercises that follow and of the Focus levels.

Response to the seminars has been very good to date, with the smallest group being forty-five and the largest 125. It is common for many to travel from afar by train, bringing blankets and food, sleeping at the seminar location overnight, just to make their attendance possible. During seminars, the participants are incredibly attentive—and also remarkably innocent.

Response to the technology itself has also been very good. Frequently, by the time we reach the *Introduction to Focus 10* exercises, there are experiences of "conscious snoring" throughout the group—a significant demonstration of the "mind awake/body asleep" state. In Wroclaw, Poland, one young lady went "out-of-body" during the very first tape exercise. She spent the remainder of the seminar trying hard to stay in! I have had many reports from participants of changes that have been effected: pill-taking insomniacs having their sleep cycle normalized after a couple of days listening to *Sleeping Through the Rain*; increased creativity; contact with inner guidance; phased "out-of-body" experiences; and even more esoteric happenings. Though I try very hard to keep their feet on the ground and emphasize the practical aspect, it can be difficult. There is so much interest in the esoteric side and many are even aware of the information in Robert Monroe's books!

I suggest to participants that they continue to practice what they have learned during the weekend. Almost all of them buy a Metamusic tape to support and enhance the process after the seminar is over.

During 1992, I returned to Budapest for a second seminar and made my first venture into Czechoslovakia. The introductory session was attended by 160 people and fifty participated in the weekend seminar, buying all the tapes I had available. Subsequently I was invited to speak at the annual Transpersonal Psychology Conference in Prague.

And how did this begin? It had very little to do with my intelligence or skill and everything to do with just being clear with "what" I want, letting go of "how" I think it should happen, and being open to what comes along. My desire was and is to assist in making the Hemi-Sync technology available to many people.

Excursion Workshops
Philip Shaffer

Phil Shaffer held a highly responsible position in NASA and now describes himself as a "consultant and investor." He has run Excursion workshops in several states in the USA.

My primary function in running workshops is to open the door for the "closet spooks" that I find around the country. It seems to me there are a great many people who have an interest in what is called the spiritual world or the metaphysical world or the New Age world, who don't know how to move out of where they are, socially or professionally, and into their own interest without causing themselves problems. People who are concerned that anyone knows they are doing this often fear they will be looked upon unfavorably.

I have found "closet spooks"—by this I mean people with an unpublicized interest in this area—everywhere, including in the ranks of the astronaut corps, aerospace engineers, farmers, physicians, psychiatrists, psychologists, teachers, and so on. What I aim to do is to introduce those people to one particular way to open the door of the closet. That, I consider, is what the expanded state of awareness is mostly about.

I use the Monroe brochure called "Are Thoughts Really Things?" to demonstrate fairly conclusively that there is some technology, there is some empirical, experiential information, that supports what it is that we are doing. That, coupled with the *Way of Hemi-Sync* tape, helps people to see that there is something valid in this. It seems to me, after three years' experience, that this also helps people to relax before a course begins.

I see problem-solving as a major item in the program, and there are specific exercises dealing with this. When we do those exercises, I advise participants not to go for big questions and big answers, such as how to solve the world's hunger problem, but to concentrate on how to frame questions, how to recognize a response of some kind, and how to learn to interpret the response. One of the innovations is encouraging people to dialogue about the response they get, either by expanding the question or clarifying the response or asking for a response in a different modality—anything that allows them to interact with whatever the source of the information is. If that is an innovation of mine, then it is one of the primary things I have brought to this practice, because if the participants go away from workshops very comfortable with framing questions in real time they have learned a skill of much value.

Here is an example from my own experience. When I took the training myself, the exercises included problem-solving in Focus 12. One of my questions was whether it was possible for me to make contact with a person I was trying to do some scheduling with. I asked the question simply—would I be able to get hold of Martha today? The response I got was a kinesthetic waffle that made no sense to me. I came back immediately with another question: "What is the meaning of this response?" This time I received a verbal answer: "It all depends. She's going out later." That was so clear that I had no reservation or hesitation about it. I called Martha early that evening and her first words were "You called just in time—I was on my way out."

That sequence of a question, followed by a lack of comprehension or a need for clarification, followed by a second question about the response, is characteristic of what I see happening in the workshops that I do. After they've done this once or twice, people become comfortable with it. Their excitement begins to grow as they get increasingly capable of framing concise questions and recognizing that a response has occurred.

I have conducted workshops in Texas, Oklahoma, California, Illinois, Florida—if we can get enough people together to pay my expenses I'll do a workshop, as it is important to me that people have access to this technology and understand what it is about and how to use it. I have introduced several innovations, including exercises to give people a little practice in experiencing and recognizing comprehension or understanding—or Aha!—whatever you want to call it, and I do that in the form of riddles. These riddles are really not designed for anybody to solve, but for people to struggle with for a while until they are struck with a sense of insight, comprehension, and release at understanding the solution. Probably the simplest one is to write on a flip chart "VII" and say "With one line, change this to an eight." Soon somebody says "Roman numeral VIII." I say, "Good," and then I write "IX" and say "With one line make this a six." They struggle for a time—and then I write "S" in front of

"IX"—and there is the "Aha!"—you see eyes broadening and quick smiles flickering. That gives me the opportunity to talk about making up rules where none were given and particularly rules that most people assume; for example, that since the first solution is a Roman numeral then the next problem is also a Roman numeral, and that they're constrained to using straight lines—I did not say anything about that.

Another example is to write two lines of letters: *A, E, F, H, I* and *B, C, D, G, J.* The problem is to determine in which group *K* goes. People look for all kinds of numerical and mathematical sequences, patterns, and so on. Then I say, "*K* goes in the top line, because the top line is made up of letters formed out of straight lines; the bottom out of letters with curved lines." It is the same thing, with the same response—they have experienced insight and comprehension.

I also emphasize that if the form or approach to anything you are using does not work, you should try a different approach. One of the other riddles I use is a number sequence: *8, 5, 4, 9, 1, 7, 6, 10, 32.* I ask, "What is the rule for ordering these numbers in this way?" People look without success for numerical sequences. Finally I say, "They are alphabetical—look at the words." You get the same physiological response. That is the point I reiterate time and again— if the approach you are using is not working, try a different approach. There is nothing sacred about the first process for solving a problem if it does not work. This carries over with some participants, helping them to adjust the way they live their lives.

One way I invite people to come to a workshop is to ask them to listen to a tape. Most naive listeners—those not specially interested in consciousness study—respond decisively. They will have a visual experience that is outside their usual orbit, or they may even feel as if they are moving out of body. One man I approached, a psychotherapist, had never heard of Hemi-Sync. He agreed to try it, as it was something new, and I sat him down to listen to *Outreach.* After about three minutes, he appeared to be in a light trance—his face was expressionless, he was completely relaxed, eyes closed and still. When the tape was over, he came back; his eyes were very wide, and I asked him what had happened. He said, "I can hear stereophonically!" I said, "That's no big deal—everybody does." He said, "You don't understand—I was hurt in a swimming accident ten years ago and I haven't been able to hear out of one ear. But now I can." I was dumbfounded. My explanation for this is that after he was healed from the injury his brain failed to reconnect the audio cross-coupling, and there was something in the Hemi-Sync experience that re-alerted him, reset him to the fact that that ear and its connectivity to the brain now worked. Alternatively it simply opened the window for a healing experience, and that is what took place. Either explanation indicates a major accomplishment for Hemi-Sync technology.

Later I did a workshop for some of his staff. Most were not initially interested but there were some "closet spooks" among them. Several had profound experiences and about half when I see them will tell me of experiences they have had since the workshop, concerning creativity or information access. They are all dialoguers, which helps them to understand responses, or why none comes.

Most of my workshops are attended by a majority who know something about states of consciousness and want to expand. For the most part, the workshop provides a different way, an optional way, to do the things they are already doing, with the additional idea of dialoguing with Source about the form or appropriateness of response. Everybody likes the experience of Hemi-Sync. In these workshops, there tends to be plenty of emotional development; the participants are quick to become involved, and what they get involved in and ask about often has an emotional signature. That seems to me very constructive; it is generally both cathartic and therapeutic.

Recently I undertook four contrasting programs. One was in western Oklahoma. It was not a big group, but to get any group in that part of the world was amazing. I had an orthodontist and his wife, a farmer and his wife, a rancher, and a bank officer. The farmer and his wife voiced some interest; they were not "closet spooks" with me but they may have been with other folks. The rest came mostly because of my reputation in the area, since it was not very far from where I had grown up and many knew of me from my time in NASA.

The first thing of note was that the rancher went into Focus 10 and enjoyed that state so much that when the exercise was over he would not come back. It occurred to me that he was in something similar to a hypnotic state. I brought him back by whispering in his ear and counting backwards, telling him that I would continue until he could not stand it any more. Eventually he came back, but it was always a struggle—he did not want to.

The bank officer had multiple sclerosis. By the end of the workshop, she was highly motivated and energized to try some alternative modalities for her condition. That was a classic case to me of opening the door for a "closet spook." She found out that there were many alternative and constructive ways which she could take advantage of. When I last saw her a few months ago, she had not deteriorated further and, more important, her attitude had greatly improved.

The farmer and his wife developed a whole new way of scheduling their activities. They owned a small retail business and had many organizational problems. They quickly discovered ways of using Focus 10 and 12 to get some insight into their difficulties. I find accessing information in Focus 10 is more effective if the information is fairly current or in the past and is quite detailed. If it is more conceptual or global, or is in the future, Focus 12 seems to work better. Suggesting this helps people to use the technology more effectively and to know which focus level to use.

The orthodontist was the biggest skeptic of the group. I suspected that his wife was a "closet spook" to everyone but him, and that it was she who had caused him to come along. During the workshop, he asked very pointed questions and was altogether cautious as to what we were doing. I tell people that as the workshop progresses the kind of information they access may become so personal they may not be comfortable in sharing it with the rest of us. When we did problem-solving in Focus 10, his presentation, demeanor, and participation changed. He began almost to withdraw from participating and became more and more reserved. Finally I asked him what was going on. His response was, "It's none of your damn business! When do we start the next exercise?" Later it transpired that what had happened was that he suddenly realized that he had access to information that he previously was ignorant of, and that some of it was extraordinary. From that point on, he was deeply immersed in learning how to use the technology, and he began interacting with us about the process and what he was doing. But he held the content close to himself, and I told him that was perfectly all right.

The second workshop was with the employees of a major aerospace firm. This group was larger and included people from senior management level, executives who had previously been engineers, down to worker-bee-level folks from the Human Resources section, and everything in between. This was an interesting group. The riddles, the "Aha's," the tape demonstration, provided enough of an ordinary reality and a technical basis for what we were about to do, and they were quickly relaxed. We did well with all the imaging exercises until we got to problem-solving. The more technical the people were, the less willing they were to acknowledge or recognize that they had received a response. They struggled to find a signature to let them know when they were in Focus 10 or 12 and seemed to accomplish that, but they believed, or appeared to believe, that Source was outside themselves, rather than accepting that Source might be their unconscious, or that their unconscious might be the gateway through which they were accessing information. We pressed on and let those who were able to access information serve as models for those who could not.

Several months later, I came across most of the participants and discovered that a higher proportion of them than was usual were still involved with the Hemi-Sync technology. They were continuing to try to learn from it and use it. For some of them it had become a normal course of their everyday business to use Focus 10 and 12 for enabling creativity when needed or for accessing information. The Human Resource employee asked me to do a workshop for the rest of his organization, as he felt he had been significantly enabled through access to this technology.

The senior manager who was present did turn out to be a "closet spook," but ended up with a conflict between the technology and his Catholic upbringing. He ultimately refused to use the processes because he thought they were in conflict with the church's teaching—the things we were doing, or talking about doing, were, he considered, reserved for the priesthood. I am still unable to persuade him otherwise. However, he is "out of the closet," but he is very restricted on what he will consider doing, although he does use Metamusic for relaxation.

The third group came with their own agenda. They wanted to establish whether changing into a different state of awareness would help them with some of their professional problems. They were introduced by an associate of mine, a psychotherapist from California, who tries to keep abreast with what is happening in her local professional community. She believed that all her colleagues had at least one patient with whom they were making no progress. She knew something of what I was doing but had no experience of work in Focus 10 and 12. When I described that, she asked me to organize a workshop to which she would bring half a dozen therapists—psychotherapists and psychiatrists—with each of them bringing one problem patient, to see if this shifting of the state of awareness on the part of either or both of the couples would provide the basis for a breakthrough.

The workshop took place a few weeks later. The patients recognized each other and the doctors all knew each other, so the patients sat together and the therapists sat together. It was hard for me to keep a straight face. The patients leapt into the technology and into the altered experience—they were more than willing to jump in. The roles were reversed, and the patients became the leaders. They were having the experiences and talking about progress and different modalities of sensory awareness, while their therapists were sitting back saying, "What happened?" The therapists began to struggle to catch up. We had two days of the patients making major breakthroughs in terms of their comprehension of what was going on and their understanding of how their mental processes did or did not fit into ordinary reality. It gave them access to their unconscious that many of them had never had before. Those who were hallucinating began to find some understanding of where the hallucinations came from and what they were about. The dynamism and energy were remarkable. The doctors never quite caught up—they were mainly locked into the constraint of "If I don't understand how it works then it cannot work." But the majority eventually did make progress and came to appreciate that "If what you're trying does not work, try something different."

Those who used the technology the most were the patients, though a couple of the doctors, including my friend, now use it as a matter of course. She is probably the only one who does so for intentional relaxation. She found it a great help in the aftermath of the Oakland earthquakes, both personally and with others—she was distributing Metamusic tapes to help people slow down and alleviate their anxiety, which they usually did.

The objectives of my workshops are to enable participants to achieve expanded states of awareness, to enhance their creativity, and to enable them to access information not normally available to them in their everyday activities. Whatever their chosen path, this technology can provide a faster way of getting where they want to go. . .and that, for the most part, is what happens.

Addenda

The Monroe Tapes

MIND FOOD SERIES

Practical Applications:

The Way of Hemi-Sync. Introduction and demonstration of the sound process.

Awake and Alert. A stimulus to stay alert.

Cable Car Ride. A music wake-up tape after tape experiences or a night's sleep.

Concentration. To enhance focus of attention. Sound signals only.

Deep 10 Relaxation. Guided imagery to reduce stress, burnout, and fatigue by attaining deep states of mental and physical relaxation.

De-Hab Smoking. Helping to break the smoking habit.

Energy Walk. A guided journey to improve strength, balance, and harmony.

Love Tennis. Visualization exercises and concentration training.

Morning Exercise. To set the tone for the day.

Nutricia. To control the body's processing of what is eaten. To improve digestion.

Pain Control. To reduce the importance of pain perception.

Retain-Recall-Release. To enable conscious control over memory.

Sound Sleeper. For a refreshing full night's sleep.

Super Sleep. For sound sleep and dream recall.

Super Senses Touch. Exploring the potentials of the sense of touch.

Surf. Sounds of ocean surf with Hemi-Sync. Helps to eliminate tension.

Under-Par Golf. Visualization and focused attention exercises.

Personal Development:

Guide to Serenity. For progressive relaxation, emotional and physical, leading into sleep.

Moment of Revelation. Aids self-understanding, tranquility, and insight by accessing higher levels of awareness.

Resonant Tuning. Breathing exercises for physical recharging, quieting the mind, and meditation.

Soft and Still. Alone with the sea and soft coastal breezes.

The Visit. A guided journey to access information and reassurance from sources other than the conscious mind.

* * * * *

THE HUMAN PLUS (H-PLUS) SERIES

Each tape carries a Prep side to explain the process, provide a relaxation technique, and establish an Access Channel. Several of the tapes are also available in French. Please note that (P) after a title indicates that the Function Command, once operational, is permanently installed; repeated use of the Function Command intensifies the effect.

Attention. To focus mind and senses on a particular thought, action, or event.

Brain: Repair & Maintenance (P). Learn to improve the blood flow, chemical and electrical activity in the brain.

Buy the Numbers (P). To help with numerical concepts and mathematical skills.

Circulation (P). To help develop smooth and optimum blood flow.

Contemplation. To facilitate a mentally active state for the inflow of ideas, intuition, and understanding.

De-Discomfort. Turns down chronic pain signals to a tolerable level.

De-Hab. For diminishing and releasing detrimental physical, emotional, or mental habits or patterns.

De-Tox: Body (P). To enhance the body's ability to cleanse itself of harmful substances.

Eat/No Eat. To help control your appetite.

Eight-Great (P). Redirect mental and physical states to express your best and inspire confidence.

Emergency: Injury. To increase natural healing and balancing abilities when physically injured.

Emergency: Toxic. To help in protecting against and discharging harmful, traumatic, or life-threatening substances.

Empathizing. To enhance understanding and sensitivity to emotional, mental, and physical states of others.

Heart: Repairs & Maintenance (P). To establish improvement in tissue functioning and blood flow of the heart.

Hypertension. A specialist tape designed to help the listener deal with blood pressure higher than normal, and any problems this may cause.

Immunizing (P). Alerting and reinforcing the immune system.

Imprint. To help achieve retention of desired information.

Let Go. To reduce or release overwhelming emotional reactions.

Light Foot. To increase efficiency of movement when walking, etc.

Lungs: Repair & Maintenance (P). Establish improvement in respiratory function.

Make Your Day. To program productive all-round daily performance.

Möbius West. To help facilitate achievement of desires or goals.

Nutricia. Learn to control your caloric intake.

Off-Loading. Release restrictive and destructive mental, emotional and physical patterns.

Options. For help in problem-solving by providing an instant overview.

Recall. For selective recall of information and experience.

Recharge. To restore physical and mental energy with brief spells of sleep.

Regenerate (P). To assist physical healing by supporting natural processes.

Relax. Gain freedom from tension while staying alert.

Release. To turn off a function currently in operation.

Reset. To restore high energy levels and change pattern from "down" to "up."

Restorative Sleep. To enhance recuperation during sleep.

See-Be. To convert any consciously controlled physical or mental activity into an automatic response.

Sensory: Hearing. To amplify or decrease your sense of hearing.

Sensory: Seeing (P). To improve and fine-tune your sense of sight.

Sensory: Smell. To amplify or decrease your sense of smell.

Sensory: Taste. To develop discrimination in taste.

Sex Drive. To increase, decrease, or re-channel sexual energy.

Short Fix. To provide immediate temporary relief from pain.

Sleep. To move easily into sleep in routine conditions.

Sleep Easy. To achieve normal sleep in non-routine or adverse circumstances.

Speak Up (P). To improve your all-round ability to speak confidently in public.

Stay Awake. To keep awake and alert when necessary in the short term.

Strong-Quick. To gain instant strength and fast reaction—short term only.

Sweet Dreams. To select dream content and remember it.

Synchronizing (P). To maximize mind/body coordination.

Think Fast (P). Speed up thought processes and reaction time.

Tune-Up. To adjust, balance, or maintain any part of the body.

Wake/Know. Make decisions and solve problems during sleep and bring information into the waking state.

Zoning. Reduce sensitivity to heat or cold.

Note: H-PLUS is a learning system and is not intended to replace conventional medical diagnosis and treatment.

TIMEOUT TAPES, SPECIFICALLY
FOR SLEEP AND REST

Catnapper. Compresses the 90-minute sleep cycle into 30 minutes. For recovery of lost sleep or jet lag.

Flying Free. A guided experience leading into dreaming sleep. Appropriate for children.

Sleepy Locust. A bedtime story for adults and children.

Deep 10 Relaxation, Surf, Sleeping Through the Rain, Sound Sleeper, and *Super Sleep* are also especially conducive to sleep.

* * * * *

PROGRESSIVE ACCELERATED LEARNING

Progressive Accelerated Learning (PAL) Albums contain exercises designed to increase the ability to focus attention and retain information.

The *Student Package* consists of the following tapes: *Concentration, Retain-Recall-Release, Awake and Alert,* and *Catnapper.*

The *Executive Package* includes the above, plus *Deep 10 Relaxation* and *Midsummer Night.*

* * * * *

Also Available:

In-Sync Golf. A compact disc designed with Hemi-Sync signals to improve your golfing performance.

METAMUSIC

Metamusic tapes are musical compositions incorporating Hemi-Sync signals which provide mental relaxation and offer unique opportunities for heightened creativity and stress reduction. The extensive list of Metamusic selections available can be obtained from The Monroe Institute.

Some Useful Books

Ash, David, and Peter Hewitt. *Science of the Gods*. Bath, England: Gateway Books, 1990.

Carter, Gari. *Healing Myself*. Norfolk, VA: Hampton Roads Publishing Company, Inc., 1993.

Hutchison, Michael. *Megabrain: New Tools and Techniques for Mind Expansion.*

Llinas, Rodolfo R. (ed). *The Workings of the Brain*. New York: Freeman & Co., 1990.

Maxwell, Meg, and Verena Tschudin. *Seeing the Invisible*. London: Arkana, 1990.

McMoneagle, Joseph. *Mind Trek*. Norfolk, VA: Hampton Roads Publishing Company, Inc., 1993.

Monroe, Robert A. *Journeys Out of the Body*. New York: Doubleday, 1972.

_____*Far Journeys*. New York: Doubleday, 1985.

_____*Ultimate Journey*. New York: Doubleday, 1994.

Ornstein, Robert, and David Sobel. *The Healing Brain*. New York: Simon & Schuster, 1988.

Ostrander, Sheila, and Lynn Schroeder. *Supermemory: The Revolution*. Carroll & Graf.

Pearce, Joseph Chilton. *Evolution's End*. San Francisco: Harper, 1992.

Russell, Peter. *The White Hole in Time*. New York: Harper Collins, 1992.

Stockton, Bayard. *Catapult: The Biography of Robert A. Monroe*. Norfolk, VA: Donning, 1988.

Talbot, Michael. *The Holographic Universe*. New York: Harper Collins, 1991.

Tart, Charles T. *States of Consciousness*. New York: Dutton, 1975.

_____ *Open Mind, Discriminating Mind*. New York: Harper Collins, 1989.

Wolman, Benjamin B., and Montague Ullman. *Handbook of States of Consciousness*, New York: Van Nostrand Rheinhold, 1986.

Useful Addresses

The Monroe Institute
Rt 1, Box 175
Faber, Virginia 22938-9749
Phone: 804-361-1252
Fax: 804-361-1237
For general inquiries, programs, details of Outreach trainers, and contacts worldwide.

Interstate Industries, Inc.
P.O. Box 505
Lovingston, Virginia 22949-0505
Phone: 804-263-8692
Fax: 804-263-8699
Credit card orders: 1-800-541-2488 (in U.S. & Canada)
For Monroe tapes and other materials.